Simply Baby:

An invaluable quick reference to infants

Megan Wissel
Joanne Smith, MD, FAAP

Dog Ear Publishing
4010 W. 86th Street, Ste H
Indianapolis, IN 46268
www.dogearpublishing.net

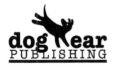

dog ear
PUBLISHING

ISBN: 978-160844-445-8
This book is printed on acid-free paper.

Disclaimer

This book serves as a basic reference guide and is not applicable to
every child in every situation. Parents and caregivers should always
follow their personal medical, legal, and financial advisors over the
advice given in this book.

The author recommends discussing all of the topics covered in this
book with the baby's pediatrician, state and local authorities, and
attorneys before implementing any practices, procedures, or advice.

Contents

1. First Days   7

FMLA	8
Breast Milk vs. Formula	10
Newborn Breast Feeding	11
Saving Cord Blood	11
Common Newborn Procedures	12
Pacifier Use	13

2. Paperwork   15

Birth Certificate	17
Social Security Card	17
Medical Insurance	18
Life Insurance	19
Wills vs. Trusts	20

3. Development   21

Growth Charts (0 to 36 months)	23
Clothing Sizing Charts	27
Development Milestones	28
Diaper Sizes	30
Promote Learning	30
Introducing New Things Calendar	31
Behavior and Discipline	32

4. Eating   33

Liquid Feeding Amounts vs. Age	35
Breast Feeding Basics	36
Breast Milk Preparation	38
Breast Milk Storage	39
Weaning from Breast Milk to Formula	40
Refusing a Bottle	40
Starting Solid Food	41
Introducing a Cup	41
Starting Finger Foods	42
Toddler Nutrition	43
Suggested Nutrition by Age	44
Vitamins, Minerals, & Nutrients Explained	45
Organic Foods	49

Contents *(cont.)*

5. Sleeping   51

Sleep Schedule Chart   53
Sleep Advice   53
Sleep Training   55
Sleeping Through the Night   57

6. Baby Sign Language   59

7. Health, Medicine, & Illness   65

Wellness Doctor Visits   67
Immunization Schedule   67
Immunization Type Explanations   68
Diseases Immunizations Protect Against   69
Bowel Movements   70
Signs of Serious Illness   71
Acetaminophen Dosage Chart   73
Ibuprofen Dosage Chart   73
Unit Conversions   74
Reducing Sickness   74
Disinfecting   75
Common Baby Illnesses and Discomforts   76
    Cold and Flu   76
    Colic   77
    Constipation   78
    Diaper Rash   79
    Diarrhea   80
    Ear Infection   81
    Fever   81
    Food Intolerance   82
    Gas & Burping   83
    Nasal Congestion   83
    Reflux   84
    Teething   85
    Vomiting   86
Probiotics   88

8. Safety & First Aid   89

SIDS (Sudden Infant Death Syndrome)   91
Child Proofing   92
House Safety   93
Out and About Safety   93
Emergency Preparedness   93
First Aid   95
    Bone Fractures   96
    Burns or Scalding   96
    Choking   97
        Choking Infants   97
        Choking Toddlers   98
    CPR (Cardiopulmonary Resuscitation) 99
        Infant CPR   100
        Toddler CPR   102
    Cuts and Scrapes   104
    Electrical Shock   104
    Foreign Object in Eye   105
    Heat Stroke   106
    Head Injuries/Trauma   106
    Insect Bites/Stings   107
    Poisoning   108
    Puncture   109
    Severe Bleeding   109
    Shock   109
    Sunburn   110
    Tick Bites   111

End Materials

Babysitter Checklist   113
Emergency Phone Numbers & Info   114

By the Author

As a mother, I can sympathize with the lack of a fast, accessible, and complete reference during situations when I need basic information. I found myself collecting notes, pamphlets, and flyers yet couldn't find what I was looking for when I had a question.

This book is designed to inform in an efficient manner, but without the detail of a technical medical text. It is not a know-it-all book and you won't find all the answers in it. It will be a valuable resource when you need to find a tidbit in a hurry and can't read pages of information. I have compiled a to-the-point reference manual for parents who have just a couple minutes, not hours, to read a chapter of information.

I hope this book serves you well. Enjoy.

– Megan Wissel

By the Contributing Editor

As a pediatrician, I receive multiple phone calls a day about routine infant and childcare. I am always happy to answer these questions, but I know many parents would like easy access to the answers themselves. This book is an excellent reference manual to inform and validate their concerns.

Have fun on the most rewarding and enjoyable adventure of your life – being a parent!

- Joanne Smith, MD, FAAP

Chapter 1

First Days

Every new parent is nervous about the delivery process and the important moments afterward. Whatever the circumstance, each and every person feels uniquely different about what they are about to experience. This chapter will hopefully ease your worries with some important information.

FMLA – FAMILY MEDICAL LEAVE ACT

Check with employer about FMLA well in advance, at least 30 days before the baby's due date and/or adoption.

US federal law provides certain protections to new parents and their jobs. Covered employers must grant an eligible employee up to a total of 12 work weeks of unpaid leave during any 12-month period for the birth and care of a newborn child of the employee, serious prenatal conditions (not routine well-visits), and for the placement with the employee of a son or daughter for adoption or foster care.

FMLA applies to all public agencies – including local, state, federal, local educational agencies, and private-sector employers who employ 50 or more employees in 20 or more work weeks in the current or preceding calendar year and who engage in commerce or activity affecting commerce – including joint employers and successors of covered employers.

In order to be covered under FMLA, an employee must:
1.) work for a covered employer,
2.) have worked for the employer for a total of 12 months,
3.) have worked at least 1250 hours of the prior 12 months, and
4.) work at a location in the United States or in any territory or possession of the United States where at least 50 employees are employed by the employer within 75 miles.

Spouses employed by the same employer are jointly entitled to a **combined** total of 12 work weeks of family leave for the birth and care of the newborn child or for the placement of a child for adoption or foster care.

Leave for birth and care, or adoption placement must conclude within 12 months of birth or placement.

Employees may take FMLA leave intermittently (taking blocks of time or reducing their normal work schedule), but it is subject to employer approval for childbirth and adoption placement.

A covered employer is required to maintain group health insurance coverage for an employee on FMLA leave whenever such insurance was provided before the leave was taken and on the same terms as if the employee had continued to work. If applicable, arrangements will need to be made for employees to pay their share of health insurance premiums while on leave. In some instances, the employer may recover premiums it paid to maintain health coverage for an employee who fails to return to work from FMLA leave.

Employers may require employees to provide:
- Medical certification supporting the need for leave due to a serious health condition affecting the employee or an immediate family member;
- Second or third medical opinions (at the employer's expense) and periodic recertification; and
- Periodic reports during FMLA leave regarding the employee's status and intent to return to work.

Covered employers must post a notice explaining rights and responsibilities under FMLA. Employers must inform employees of their rights and responsibilities under FMLA, including giving specific written information on what is required of the employee and what might happen in certain circumstances, such as if the employee fails to return to work after FMLA leave. It is unlawful for any employer to interfere with, restrain, or deny the exercise of any right provided by FMLA. It is also unlawful for an employer to discharge or discriminate against any individual for opposing any practice, or because of involvement in any proceeding, related to FMLA.

Only the FMLA information regarding prenatal, childbirth, and adoption is listed. For more information and questions, contact employer and/or:

Wage and Hour Division of the US Department of Labor
http://www.wagehour.dol.gov
1-866-4USWAGE (1-866-487-9243)

BREAST MILK VS. FORMULA

The longer an infant is breast fed, the better, up to 12 months of age. Every family and every mother is different and the general consensus is to breast feed as long as the mother is able. The advantages and disadvantages of breast feeding are below.

BREAST FEEDING ADVANTAGES

- **Reduced Illness** – Breast fed babies are sick less often because of the antibodies found in breast milk. Antibodies may reduce ear infections, diarrhea, respiratory infections, meningitis, allergies, diabetes, and SIDS (Sudden Infant Death Syndrome).
- **Nutrition** – Breast milk has all the necessary nutrients for an infant with the exception of Vitamin D. Breast milk has complex substances that are too difficult to manufacture and some have not yet been identified.
- **Ease of Digestion** - Breast fed babies tend to have fewer digestive problems, such as spit-up or irregular bowls.
- **Different Tastes** – When a mother consumes different foods, the taste passes to the breast milk and better prepares the baby for the variety of flavors solid foods offer.
- **Convenience** – Breast milk is always available and ready to consume. There are no bottles to wash/sanitize or formula to buy at the store.
- **Obesity Prevention** – The National Women's Health Information Center (part of the U.S. Department of Health and Human Services) states that babies who are breast fed tend to gain less unnecessary weight, which may help avoid obesity later.
- **Smarter Child** – Some recent research states that infants exclusively breast fed for six months scored five to ten points higher on IQ tests.
- **Cost** – Breast milk is free, while formula can be very expensive at more than $120 per month.
- **Content and Volume Changes** - Based on age and demand of baby. At different ages, the infant receives different nutrient combinations to best fit what the infant needs.
- **Mother's Health** – Breast feeding requires up to 500 calories a day to produce, aiding the loss of pregnancy weight. Nursing also speeds uterus contraction, and may decrease the risk of anemia, post-menopausal breast cancer, uterine cancer, and ovarian cancer.

BREAST FEEDING DISADVANTAGES
- **Mother's Comfort**- Breast feeding may hurt when the baby is not properly latched on. This can cause cracked nipples that can be painful.
- **Mother's Schedule** – Breast feeding can take time.
- **Mother's Diet**- While breast feeding, mothers should limit their caffeine and alcohol intake, take prenatal vitamins, and be sure to eat properly.

NEWBORN BREAST FEEDING
The American Academy of Pediatrics suggests breast feeding a minimum of six months. The first few days and weeks are critical because the antibodies in breast milk help the undeveloped immune system.
- Breast feed as soon as possible after delivery.
- If the baby isn't nursing successfully within 3-4 hours, discuss pumping options with a nurse or lactation consultant.
- Do not give a newborn a bottle (even with expressed milk), or a pacifier until breast feeding is established, usually by 2-3 weeks. This can cause nursing problems even in babies who are successful nursers.

See Breast Feeding Basics section in the Eating Chapter.

SAVING CORD BLOOD
Blood rich in stem cells unique to a baby can be collected from the umbilical cord right after giving birth. This is a family decision and is very costly (over $1,000). Stem cells are unique to any other cell because they can transform into any other type of body cell.

Families choose to save cord blood, often called cord blood banking, for future potential medical reasons including life-threatening diseases. The cord blood has stem cells, which may be used to treat many medical problems such as leukemia, heart disease, strokes, and Alzheimer's.

Cord blood is very easily collected after the umbilical cord has been clamped and cut without any disruption to the baby or mother. Once collected, it goes to a processing facility and is stored in liquid nitrogen. If parents do not choose to save their newborn's cord blood, it will be discarded by the hospital.

COMMON NEWBORN PROCEDURES

Newborns undergo a variety of tests while in the hospital. Each state has different laws for mandatory screening/testing done on newborns.

- **Apgar Score** – Test taken at one minute and five minutes after birth with scores from 0-10. The doctor or nurse rates the following on a scale of zero to two to arrive at a total score: activity and muscle tone, pulse, reflex irritability (grimace response), skin appearance, and breathing rate.

- **Hearing Tests** - Baby will most likely have one of the following that determines if hearing nerves are present; these are not absolute tests that determine normal hearing levels.

  - **ABR** – Auditory Brainstem Response: This tests the integrity of the hearing system to the brain, which is measured by placing four or five electrodes on the forehead introducing a variety of sounds via earphones.

  - **OAE** – OtoAcoustic Emissions: This test measures the acoustic response that is delivered by the inner ear, or cochlea. The infant will be resting when a probe, which has a microphone and speaker, is placed in the ear. The speaker generates a small noise and the microphone measures the sound generated by the inner ear.

- **Erythromycin Ointment or Silver Nitrate** – This is placed in a newborn's eyes for protection from eye diseases.

- **Vitamin K** – Some newborns are born with a vitamin K deficiency, which can cause bleeding within the brain. Vitamin K, which promotes blood clotting, is injected as a precaution for this condition.

- **NBS** – This is short for a NewBorn Screen; it is sometimes called a "heel prick" or "PKU" test. Several drops of blood will be taken from the newborn's heel at 48 to 72 hours after birth to test for genetic abnormalities and other diseases. The diseases that will be tested for depend on the state where the baby was delivered.

- **Hepatitis B** – This is hospital dependent and requires parent's consent. This is the first vaccine to protect against Hepatitis B.

- **Bilirubin** – In most hospitals, a bilirubin level is routinely checked greater than 24 hours old to evaluate for jaundice. Scanning the forehead to measure the amount through the skin or through a blood test can check the bilirubin level. About 50% of newborns have at least some jaundice. High bilirubin levels are serious because they can damage the brain causing mental retardation, learning disabilities, hearing loss, or eye movement problems.

PACIFIER USE

Use of a pacifier is a personal decision.

Some points:

- Helps newborns with non-nutritive sucking desire and will calm
- A preventive device for SIDS
- If formula feeding, can start immediately at birth
- If breast feeding, can start when breast feeding is established (around 2-3 weeks)
- When 6 months of age, limit to only when sleeping
- Past 12-13 months of age, difficulty weaning will sharply increase with age

PERSONAL NOTES

Chapter 2

Paperwork

Plenty goes along with a baby other than cute outfits and bottles. This chapter describes important legal and insurance issues that go along with this new family addition.

PERSONAL NOTES

Simply Baby: An invaluable quick reference to infants

BIRTH CERTIFICATE

The county government where the child was born distributes birth certificates. The hospital will likely give parents the information to obtain a birth certificate.

Parents must contact the local county health or vital records department for more information because birth certificates are not automatic.

SOCIAL SECURITY CARD

A baby will need a social security number to be a listed dependent on parents' income taxes, get a job, collect social security benefits, and receive some other government services.

Some hospitals submit the necessary documents for newborns to receive their social security card. If the hospital did not provide this service, or Baby was not delivered in a hospital it is easy to obtain one for a child or children.

Parents or guardians will need to:
1.) Fill out an Application for a Social Security Card (Form SS-5),
2.) Show documents providing child's current citizenship, age and identity preferably with a photo and with parent's name(s), examples could include:
   a. State issued identification card
   b. Adoption decree
   c. Doctor, clinic, or hospital record
   d. Religious record
   e. Daycare center or school record
   f. School identification card,
3.) Parent's or guardian's personal proof of identity, examples can be:
   a. U.S. drivers license or non-driver identification card
   b. U.S. passport, and
4.) Take or mail all documents to local social security office.

More information at **http://www.ssa.gov/** or call **800-772-1213**

MEDICAL INSURANCE

It is crucial to have medical insurance for children. Some uninsured families cannot recover from the financial burden of a major medical emergency and end up sacrificing their status of living. If the parent's employer does not provide insurance, seek an independent source.

Whatever insurance provider, contact them before and/or immediately after the baby's birth to assure coverage. All insurance companies require parents to contact them within 30 days of the birth date.

Most medical facilities have applications for hardship in the form of charity or will discount for self-payment if asked.

Private Insurance: PPO vs. HMO Plans

HMO stands for Health Maintenance Organization. PPO stands for Preferred Provider Organization. Usually PPO plans are much less restrictive, however they require higher premiums. HMO plans are more restrictive, usually mandating that one doctor within the organization manages your healthcare.

Be sure to understand the differences and ask questions.

Medicaid

Medicaid is a state sponsored health program available to low-income families who meet the guidelines issued by their state of residence. Each state's program has a different name and different application criteria. Call 1-877-KIDS-NOW (1-877-543-7669) to learn about any state's Medicaid program. Even if guardians do not qualify for Medicaid, they still may qualify for other state programs.

Cimply Baby: An invaluable quick reference to infants

LIFE INSURANCE

Life insurance serves one purpose: to financially secure the family members of the insured if he or she were to die.

When thinking about life insurance, **each parent** must be covered. When thinking about the best premiums and payoff amounts, the following should be considered for each parent's insurance policy:

- Income loss of possible deceased parent
- Added day care expenses
- Family medical insurance premiums
- Funeral expenses
- Mortgage payoff

Items to consider if family can afford added monthly premiums to benefit:

- College expenses for children
- All personal debt payoff (i.e. credit cards, medical bills, personal loans)
- Supplement retirement contributions of possible deceased

Life insurance coverage on infants needs only to cover funeral expenses and any outstanding medical bills since the infant never contributed to the family financially.

Whole vs. term life insurance

The two main types of life insurance are whole and term policies. In a whole life policy, a person pays a small monthly or yearly premium for their entire life, with a low payout upon death (usually from $5,000 to $50,000), but a balance that increases similar to a savings account if a death benefit is not paid. In a term life policy, a person pays a monthly or yearly premium for a set term (5 to 25 years), with usually a much larger payout (usually $25,000 to +$1,000,000), but no cash surrender value. Term life insurance premiums have become more competitive recently, challenging the traditional value of the whole life policy. It is wise to get quotes on both types of policies and understand where they differ.

TRUSTS VS. WILLS

There are two types of legal documents one may and should produce to make sure his or her wishes are carried out after he or she dies. Without the necessary documents, the court system assigns a deceased parent's children and assets as it sees fit through probate. In some US states, if a living spouse exists the probate process does not take place.

The following chart outlines the basic differences in a living trust and a last will. Advisors suggest it is better to have both. A living trust is designed for titled property transfers to beneficiary to avoid the probate fees and extended process. A last will should include your children's future guardians, non-titled items (jewelry, furniture, grandpa's watch, etc.), and funeral/burial arrangements and will be subject to the probate process.

Living Trust	Last Will
Cannot name future guardians of children	Can name future guardians of children
Distributes property to beneficiaries	Distributes property to beneficiaries
May reduce estate taxes	Can specify funeral and burial arrangements
Keeps estate details private	Makes estate details public
More expensive to have drawn up	Less expensive to have drawn up
Does not go through probate - no court, executor or lawyer fees	Goes through probate - estate will pay all court, executor and lawyer fees
Much less time to execute, immediate transfer to beneficiaries	Probate process can take months, even years

Chapter 3

Development

A parent may often wonder if their child is growing and developing as they should. Every child is different and unique and will develop at his or her own pace. Three things can alter a children's growth: genetic potential, nutrition, and medical problems.

Premature babies have catching up to do and parents should use the Expected Due Date as the birth date for comparison.

PERSONAL NOTES

GROWTH CHARTS

These diagrams show boys and girls growth national percentiles from birth to 36 months of age.

Boys Length-for-age and Weight-for-age percentiles

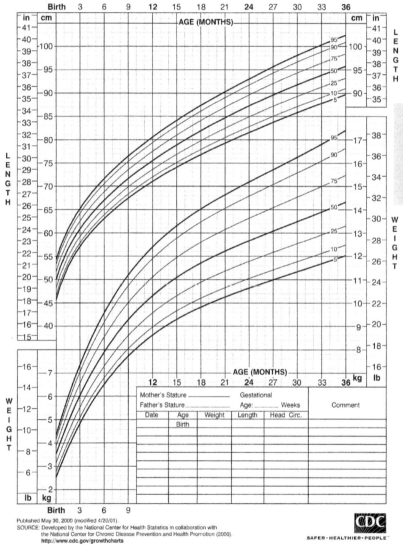

Published May 30, 2000 (modified 4/20/01).
SOURCE: Developed by the National Center for Health Statistics in collaboration with the National Center for Chronic Disease Prevention and Health Promotion (2000).
http://www.cdc.gov/growthcharts

CDC
SAFER · HEALTHIER · PEOPLE™

Development

Boys Head Circumference-for-age and Weight-for-length percentiles

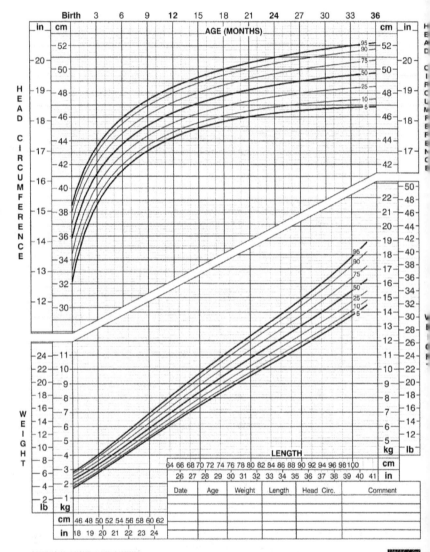

Published May 30, 2000 (modified 10/16/00).
SOURCE: Developed by the National Center for Health Statistics in collaboration with
the National Center for Chronic Disease Prevention and Health Promotion (2000).
http://www.cdc.gov/growthcharts

SAFER · HEALTHIER · PEOPLE™

Girls Length-for-age and Weight-for-age percentiles

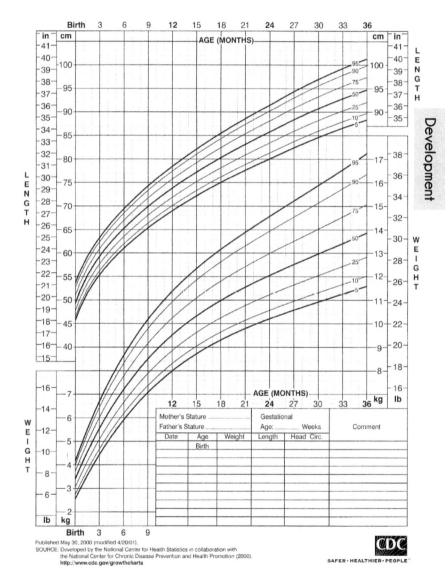

Published May 30, 2000 (modified 4/20/01).
SOURCE: Developed by the National Center for Health Statistics in collaboration with
the National Center for Chronic Disease Prevention and Health Promotion (2000).
http://www.cdc.gov/growthcharts

CDC
SAFER · HEALTHIER · PEOPLE

Girls Head Circumference-for-age and Weight-for-length percentiles

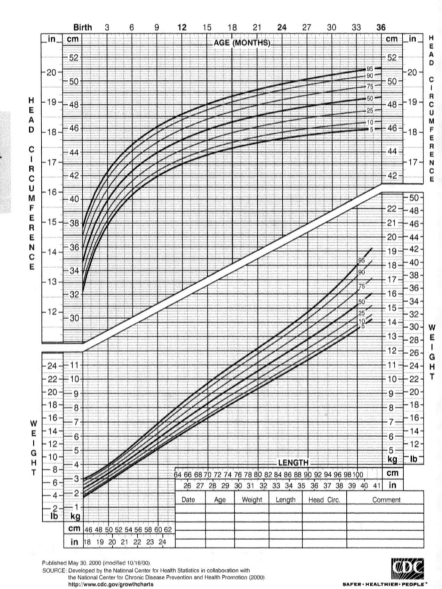

Published May 30, 2000 (modified 10/16/00).
SOURCE: Developed by the National Center for Health Statistics in collaboration with
the National Center for Chronic Disease Prevention and Health Promotion (2000).
http://www.cdc.gov/growthcharts

CDC
SAFER · HEALTHIER · PEOPLE™

SIZING CHARTS

Every brand of baby clothing may have different sizing charts for infants and toddlers, so be sure to check before buying. The chart below shows some popular brands to demonstrate the size differences and should just serve as a reference. There are also spots to fill in additional preferred clothing brands not already included.

Size	Carter's® Weight (lbs)	Carter's® Height (in)	Children's Place® Weight (lbs)	Children's Place® Height (in)	Gap®, Old Navy® Weight (lbs)	Gap®, Old Navy® Height (in)	Gerber® Weight (lbs)	Gerber® Height (in)
Newborn	5-8	17-21"			<7	<17/18"		
0-3 mths	8-12	21-24"	7-11	18-22"	7-12	17-23"	0-6	10-16"
3-6 mths	12-16	24-26"	11-15	22-25"	12-17	23-27"	7-15	17-24"
6-9 mths	16-20	26-28"	15-18	25-27"				
9-12 mths	20-24	28-30"	18-22	27-29"				
6-12 mths					17-22	27-29"	16-22	25-28"
12-18 mths	24-27	30-32"	22-26	29-31"	22-27	29-31"	23-27	29-31"
18-24 mths	27-30	32-34"			27-30	31-33"	28-30	32-34"
2T	29-31	34-36"	26-29	31-34"	30-33	33-36"		
3T	31-34	36-38"	29-32	34-37"	33-36	36-39"		

Size	Gymboree® Weight (lbs)	Gymboree® Height (in)	OshKosh® Weight (lbs)	OshKosh® Height (in)	Weight (lbs)	Height (in)	Weight (lbs)	Height (in)
Newborn	<7	<19"						
0-3 mths	7-12	<23"	5-12	20-23"				
3-6 mths	12-17	23-25"	12-16	24-26"				
6-9 mths			16-18	27-28"				
9-12 mths			18-20	29-30"				
6-12 mths	17-22	25-29"						
12-18 mths	22-27	29-31"	20-24	20-24"				
18-24 mths	27-30	31-33"	24-27	24-27"				
2T	30-32	33-36"	25-28	33-35"				
3T	32-35	36-39"	29-32	36-38"				

Development

DEVELOPMENT MILESTONES

Different babies develop at different rates; never compare babies. These milestones are a list of what many babies can do at these ages; it is normal if a baby excels in one area and is "behind" in another. If baby does not show any signs of progress or something doesn't seem quite right, discuss with the pediatrician.

1 MONTH OLD
- Begins to smile
- Makes noises other than crying
- Brings hands near face
- Moves head side to side while lying on stomach
- Prefers human faces over other objects

2 MONTHS OLD
- Smiles socially
- Focuses on objects across the room
- Raises and supports head and chest while on stomach with arms

4 MONTHS OLD
- Grabs and shakes hand toys
- Opens and shuts hands
- Brings hands to mouth
- Follows a moving object with eyes
- Enjoys playing and may cry when playing stops
- Stretches and kicks legs when on back or stomach
- Starts using hands and eyes in coordination
- Reaches for objects with one hand
- Puts objects in mouth
- Makes eye contact
- Sits with support

6 MONTHS OLD
- Rolls over both ways
- Develops adult color and distance vision
- Explores objects with mouth and hands
- Transfers objects from one hand to another
- Uses voice to express happiness or displeasure
- Starts to babble
- Blows "raspberries"
- Sits with assistance or for very short amounts of time

9 MONTHS OLD
- Supports own weight on legs when held upright
- Transfers objects from one hand to another
- Uses voice to express happiness or displeasure
- Starts to babble consonants (baba, dada, mama)
- Develops pincher grasp with two fingers
- Waves
- Claps hands
- Drinks from a cup

12 MONTHS OLD
- Sits without assistance
- Crawls
- Pulls self up to stand
- Walks holding on to furniture
- Tries imitating words and sounds
- Shakes head "no" and waves "bye"
- Explores objects in different ways, not just orally
- Looks at correct picture when object is named
- Points at objects

18 MONTHS OLD
- Says at least 15 single words
- Turns pages in a book
- Gestures and points to objects that he or she wants
- Stands alone and can walk
- Looks for objects out of sight
- Likes to take things apart
- Hands objects to others
- Plays alone on floor with toys
- Imitates others by coughing, laughing, or animal sounds
- Looks at the person talking to her or him

24 MONTHS OLD
- Scribbles with crayons
- Walks alone, begins to run, and can carry items
- Pulls and pushes wheeled toys
- Kicks a ball
- Climbs on and off furniture without assistance
- Uses simple phrases "need drink" or "want up/down"
- Follows simple instructions
- Imitates behaviors of others
- Walks up and down stairs while holding a support

Development

DIAPER SIZES

There are many brands of disposable diapers, including store brands, but the mainstream brands are Pampers®, Huggies®, and Luvs®. The different sizes of the major brands are all the same, although one diaper brand may fit your baby's body shape better than another at various stages.

Newborn	up to 10 lbs
Size 1	8-14 lbs
Size 2	12-18 lbs
Size 3	16-28 lbs
Size 4	22-37 lbs
Size 5	27 lbs +
Size 6	35 lbs +

Expect to go through 8-10 diapers a day the first few weeks after birth.

PROMOTE LEARNING

Things parents and caregivers can do at any age to promote learning:

- Read books together for at least 10-15 minutes a day.
- Narrate what is happening or being done. Such as "going up the stairs", "mommy's cleaning the dishes", "the dog is chewing on the bone", "we are getting Baby dressed, right leg in, left leg in", etc.
- When crawling and exploring, put items inside or behind other objects so Baby can "find".
- Talk and sing directly to Baby whenever possible.
- Encourage and give verbal rewards such as "good job", "what a smart baby", and "way to go" when they are doing activities.
- Never use baby talk, always speak clearly. Instead, voice tone and volume should be used for softness.
- Limit TV watching to 30 minutes per day, especially until 2 years of age.

NEW THINGS CALENDAR

Light Gray: introduction time   **Dark Gray**: should be learning
Black: should have mastered   **X**: should take place

Column labels (left to right): Potty Training · Sign Language · No bottles · Coloring Books & Crayons · Own Spoon & Fork · Own Dish (not highchair tray) · Pillow/Blanket in Crib · Dentist Visit · Walking · Standing Alone · Attachment Object · Drinking from Straw · Cup · Finger Foods · Infant Cereal & Baby Food · Crawling · Set sleep schedule · Doctor well visits

Month	Doctor well visits (X)
1 month	x
2 months	x
4 months	x
6 months	x
7 months	
8 months	
9 months	x
10 months	
11 months	
12 months	x
13 months	
14 months	
15 months	x
16 months	
17 months	
18 months	x
24 months	x
30 months	
36 months	x

BEHAVIOR AND DISCIPLINE

The different stages of development require different discipline strategies and techniques.

CRAWLING (~6-13 months old)
- Prevent problems by removing hazards from view or access
- Behavior boundaries must be set
- Limit the word "no" and redirect attention instead
- Never spank, hit, or give a "time out" to a child at this age – they do not understand

WALKING (~13-17 months old)
- Start encouraging please and thank you
- Still limit "no" and redirect when possible
- Reward good behavior
- Never spank, hit, or give a "time out" to a child at this age

TALKING and UNDERSTANDING (~17 months old or older)
- Encourage please and thank you and other manners such as sharing
- Start introducing table manners
- Redirect when possible
- Never allow tantrums or give in to tantrums, ignore them until the tantrum is finished and try to redirect attention
- Reward good behavior
- Hitting or biting should be a "no"
- Starts understanding "hot" or danger items; explain why toddler has that limit ("no" the stove is hot, or "no" it will hurt you and make an ouchy)

Chapter 4

Eating

This chapter will provide parents typical eating habits for infants and toddlers along with nutritional information.

PERSONAL NOTES

Eating

LIQUID FEEDING AMOUNTS AND SCHEDULE VS. AGE

Each baby has his or her own nutritional needs. Unless the pediatrician specifies a change, a parent should not alter feeding habits for a child that is eating regularly and gaining weight. The table below displays typical feeding habits for infants as they age.

| Age | Breast Milk or Formula Amounts | | | Allowable amount of juice or water in 24 hours |
	Average # of feedings in 24 hours	Average amount per feeding	Average amount per day	
1-2 weeks	6-10	2-3 fl oz	12-30 fl oz	0 fl oz
3-4 weeks	6-8	3-4 fl oz	18-32 fl oz	0 fl oz
1-2 months	5-6	4-5 fl oz	20-30 fl oz	0 fl oz
2-3 months	5-6	5-6 fl oz	25-36 fl oz	0 fl oz
3-4 months	4-5	6-7 fl oz	24-36 fl oz	0 fl oz
4-7 months	4-5	7-8 fl oz	28-40 fl oz	0 fl oz
7-9 months	3-4	7-8 fl oz	21-32 fl oz	2-4 oz
9-12 months	3	7-8 fl oz	21-24 fl oz	4-6 oz
12-24 months	4-6 whole milk	-	15-20 oz	4-6 oz

Eating

BREAST FEEDING BASICS

The American Academy of Pediatrics suggests breast feeding a minimum of six months. Every family and every mother is different and the general consensus is to breast feed as long as the mother is able.

Important facts and wisdom:

- Breast feed as soon as possible after delivery.
- Colostrum is released only in the first 2-3 days after delivery. This high caloric liquid has important antibodies vital to a newborn's health.
- If the baby isn't "getting it", try it again and again and again. After a few hours, ask the nurse about a lactation consultant and/or pumping options. Pumping is crucial for a mother's body to produce colostrum and later, milk.
- If nursing hurts past 20-30 seconds, the baby is not latched on correctly; reposition until it doesn't hurt. Incorrect positioning can lead to sore and chapped nipples.
- Nursing sessions should not exceed 45 minutes in the first two weeks or 30 minutes after three weeks.
- Do not let the baby feed more often than once every 2 hours after birth, every 2-1/2 hours from 1-3 months, or every 3 hours older than 3 months of age. Nursing more frequently or longer doesn't mean the baby is drinking or getting more milk. Some babies like breast feeding for comfort; mothers can show comfort and assurance by holding, cuddling, and singing instead. A mother's body needs that resting time to produce the higher nutritional milk.
- Do not give a newborn a bottle (even with expressed breast milk) or a pacifier until breast feeding is established, usually by 2-3 weeks. This can cause nursing problems even in babies who are successful nursers.
- Introduce a bottle of pumped breast milk at around 1 month of age and give expressed milk at least once a week after if planning to bottle feed later. Most breast fed babies greater than 3 months old will not take a bottle if they have not been introduced before.
- Milk is produced to match the baby's consumption. It is common for a newborn to only accept up to 2 oz of milk at the beginning, while months later drinking 8 oz or more. The exact quantity consumed and duration of nursing sessions is not as important as long as the baby is gaining weight, developing, and producing the appropriate amount of soiled diapers for their age.

- Supplemental pumping will increase milk supply. Immediately following a feeding, pump 3-5 minutes after breasts are empty. This will stimulate the mother's body to supply more milk for subsequent feedings.
- Pediatricians usually recommend breast fed babies receive Vitamin D supplement drops. Discuss with baby's pediatrician.

Nursing problems:
- Cracked nipples and/or blisters are a result of improper latching of the baby. Use of expressed breast milk, lanolin ointment, or hydro gel pads can soothe.
- Clogged milk ducts can be extremely painful. Baby must continue to feed on hurt breast. This is the only way to relieve and reduce the pressure. Use ice packs and massage to relieve soreness. Hot showers do not give relief and may cause more pain.
- If a mother gets sick, she almost always can still breast feed. The mother should point out to her doctor that she is breast feeding so any prescriptions can be altered.

Eating

BREAST MILK PREPARATION

If a mother pumps milk instead of nursing directly, this section contains guidelines on handling and preparation.

- Wash hands thoroughly before expressing or handling.
- Before collection, wash proper containers. Do not use ordinary plastic storage bags or formula bottle bags as they could spill or leak. Instead, use bags and containers especially designed for breast milk storage.
- Label milk with date it was expressed, to facilitate using the oldest milk first. If milk is going to a child-care provider, clearly label the container with child's name.
- Refrigerate or freeze milk as soon as possible if not giving immediately.
- Do not add fresh milk to already frozen milk within a storage container.
- Discard milk used from a bottle, do not use for another feeding.

IF FROZEN:
- Thaw frozen breast milk by transferring it to the refrigerator or by swirling it in a bowl of warm water.
- Do not use microwave ovens to thaw or heat bottles. They can heat unevenly easily scalding the baby and it degrades the nutrient quality of the milk.
- Do not re-freeze once thawed.

Eating

BREAST MILK STORAGE

This chart is for typical healthy infants, unless a doctor specifies otherwise.

Location	Temperature	Duration	Comments
Countertop / table	Room temperature (up to 77°F or 25°C)	6–8 hours	Containers should be covered and kept as cool as possible; covering the container with a cool towel may keep milk cooler.
Insulated cooler bag	5-39°F or -15-4°C	24 hours	Keep ice packs in contact with milk containers at all times, limit opening cooler bag.
Refrigerator	39°F or 4°C	5 days	Store milk in the back of the main body of the refrigerator.
Freezer compartment of a refrigerator	5°F or -15°C	2 weeks	Store milk toward the back of the freezer, where temperature is most constant. Milk stored for longer durations in the ranges listed is safe, but some of the lipids in the milk undergo degradation resulting in lower quality.
Freezer compartment of refrigerator with separate doors	0°F or -18°C	3–6 months	
Chest or upright deep freezer	-4°F or -20°C	6–12 months	

Eating

WEANING FROM BREAST MILK TO FORMULA

1.) Start with one bottle of formula once a day for a few days. Some infants, especially infants older than 5-6 months, will not take formula the first time because it tastes bitter or metallic compared to breast milk; breast milk can be mixed with formula (half and half) to help.

- Usually the easiest feeding to substitute first is one of the middle of the day feedings. Night feedings or a bedtime feeding should be reserved for last in the substitution sequence.

2.) Once the baby accepts formula, every other day substitute a breast fed feeding for a formula feeding.

3.) The longer the infant receives any amount of breast milk the better (less than 2 years of age). Keeping one or two breast milk feeding(s) a day (morning or evening) for a few months is very acceptable and encouraged.

If 12 months of age or older, weaning should be done straight from the breast to whole cow's milk in a cup. A bottle should not be introduced or continued.

NOTE: If the infant has never been given a bottle and they are older than 6 months old, weaning can be extremely difficult. Infants will need to learn how to suck on a bottle and they will not like the taste of what they receive. To avoid this, breast fed babies starting at one month of age should be given at least one bottle every week of expressed milk to allow them to learn and accept a bottle.

REFUSING A BOTTLE

Some breast fed infants will refuse a bottle. Some things to try:

- Larger, smaller, and different types of bottle nipples
- Different temperatures
- Someone other than mother to give bottle, if possible
- Try bottle for 15-20 minutes before every feeding before nursing until successful
- If trying with only formula in bottle, try breast milk first. After successful on breast milk, start a mixture of prepared formula and breast milk until ratio of prepared formula is 100% of mixture.

NOTE: Once a bottle has been accepted, a bottle should be given at least every 7 days thereafter to eliminate future refusal.

STARTING SOLID FOODS

Near 6 months of age, babies are ready for more than just breast milk or formula.

1.) Start with 2 tablespoons of infant iron-fortified rice cereal once a day for at least three consecutive days, mixed with breast milk or formula.
2.) Try cereals other than rice, but allow three days for any allergies to be identified and isolated.
3.) Start introduction of single vegetables and fruits that are strained and mashed one at a time.
4.) Baby should be given every new food for three consecutive days to isolate allergens.

NOTE: Try feeding baby at least one hour before or after breast milk or formula so baby is interested. (Not too full or too hungry)

INTRODUCING A CUP

- At 6-7 months of age, parents can introduce a "sippy" cup. Some infants do not take well to the cup, but try and try again. Parents can try using a regular cup, taking the valve out, or using a straw.
- Around 10-12 months of age, start eliminating bottles progressively during feedings, substituting with a cup.
  - Trying to eliminate bottles past that age can be done but it is more difficult.
  - Parents can start with removing one bottle every few days or one every week, leaving the night bottle for last.
  - Since they may not drink very much at a sitting (only an ounce or two), a cup must be offered at least 2-3 times more frequently than the bottle.
  - Bottles should be eliminated by 15 months of age because toddlers grow very attached, refusing cups and demanding bottles. Tantrums and screaming are likely past 16 months of age.
- At around 14-15 months of age, toddlers become very attached to bottles and "sippy" cups.
  - They will try to take them everywhere.
  - Starting at an early age, drinking allowed with certain boundaries - such as only while sitting or only on hard floors - will avoid messes and unnecessary attachments.

Eating

STARTING FINGER FOODS

By 7-9 months of age, a baby has developed enough coordination to start finger foods. Always feed a baby while they are sitting, strapped in, and supervised at all times.

Good starting finger foods:
- Bananas
- Round oat cereal
- Animal crackers
- Steamed diced vegetables such as carrots, green beans
- Diced cooked or canned peaches, pears
- Canned mandarin oranges
- White rice
- Beans of any variety
- Ground meat and lunch meat
- Diced and peeled baked potato
- Small cubed soft cheese: American, Swiss, mozzarella
- Toast, since soft bread can ball up in mouth and cause choking
- Well cooked pasta noodles
- Quartered and peeled grapes
- Graham crackers

Do not feed baby foods high in sodium or processed sugar.

 Foods to avoid until 12 months of age or later:
- Eggs
- Honey
- Peanut Butter (longer if a family allergy exists)
- Seafood and fish
- Cow's milk (Give whole milk from 12 months to 2 years old)

TODDLER NUTRITION

At 12 months of age, a toddler can eat whatever is served at the family table that can be easily mashed between fingers. Avoid common choking foods such as: uncut hotdogs, uncut grapes, steak, peanuts, apples, bacon, raisins, chips, popcorn, and hard candy. When feeding a toddler over 12 months old, be sure to promote healthy eating habits.

- Offer five fruit and vegetable servings a day. Serving size is ¼ cup.
- Serve whole grain cereals and breads for fiber content, approximately 2 ounces per day.
- Give healthy sources of protein such as lean meat, eggs, and soft cheese, approximately 1-2 ounces per day.
- Limit junk food, fast food, processed sugar, and high-sodium foods.
- Do not give sugary fruit drinks or soda; instead, offer water and whole milk. Allow no more than 4-6 oz. of 100% juice a day.
- Limit fried foods; bake, broil, grill, or steam when possible.

Some things to remember:
- By the age of 12 months, toddlers need three meals and two snacks a day.
- It can take up to 10 tries of a new food for a toddler to accept it.
- Don't ever force a toddler to eat; they will eat if they are hungry. Try offering something else instead or waiting 30 minutes.
- They may not want to sit in a highchair for the duration of the meal, but it is important to learn patience and a ritual location (at the table in their chair) is where they eat.
- Limit drinking and eating to times when sitting.
- Make every meal and snack time social by sitting with toddlers while they are eating for at least a few minutes. If a toddler is especially picky, have (or pretend to have) a snack or meal at the same time. Toddlers learn proper eating habits by imitation.
- Toddlers can be very finicky eaters. There are over-the-counter vitamin drops that can be added to foods or drinks. Do not rely on these supplements in a toddler's diet because natural sources are better and they do not promote healthy eating habits.

Eating

SUGGESTED NUTRITION BY AGE CHART

	0-6 months	7-12 months	1-3 yrs
Calories per pound per day	49 cal/lb	44 cal/lb	48 cal/lb
Carbohydrate (g/day)	60	95	130
Total Fiber (g/day)	ND	ND	19
Fat (g/day)	31	30	ND
Protein (g/kg/day)	1.52	1.05	0.95
Vitamin C (mg/day)	40	50	15
Vitamin D (ug/day)	5	5	5
Calcium (g/day)	210	270	500
Iron (mg/day)	0.27	11	7
Zinc (mg/day)	2	3	3
Potassium (g/day)	0.4	0.7	3
Sodium (g/day)	0.12	0.37	1

*Source of Information: *Pediatric Nutrition Handbook*, 6th Edition by the American Academy of Pediatrics Committee on Nutrition, Edited by Ronald E. Kleinman, MD, FAAP, 2009

Eating

VITAMINS, MINERALS, & NUTRIENTS EXPLAINED

Parents understand vitamins and minerals are crucial to a child's growth and development. However, some parents do not know what roles each vitamin or mineral plays or what foods have them.

Vitamins

There are two types of vitamins: water-soluble and fat-soluble. Water-soluble vitamins cannot be stored by the body and need to be replenished daily. Fat-soluble vitamins are absorbed through the intestines with the help of lipids (fats) and are stored by the body.

Vitamins taken in excess can lead to vitamin poisoning, most commonly A and D. Upper limit daily intake amounts are especially important in fat-soluble vitamins because they can accumulate in the body. Upper limits are not given in this book but can be readily acquired through various sources, including a pediatrician.

Water-Soluble Vitamins
- Vitamin B1 (Thiamin)
- Vitamin B2 (Riboflavin)
- Vitamin B3 (Niacin)
- Vitamin B5 (Pantothenic Acid)
- Vitamin B6 (Pyridoxine)
- Vitamin B9 (Folate/Folic Acid)
- Vitamin B12 (Cobalamin, Cy)
- Vitamin C (Ascorbic Acid)
- Vitamin H (Biotin)

Fat-Soluble Vitamins
- Vitamin A (Beta Carotene)
- Vitamin D
- Vitamin E
- Vitamin K

DHA (Docosahexaenoic acid) and ARA (Arachidonic acid)

DHA and ARA are naturally found in breast milk and are a type of lipid (fat). These are sometimes added to infant formula and food to promote healthy eye and brain development. The DHA and ARA lipids that are found in breast milk are structurally different than those found in infant formula or food additives. The man-made lipids are extracted from laboratory-grown fermented algae and fungus and artificially processed. Short and long term benefits of man-made lipids are non-conclusive.

Fiber

Fiber is very important for digestion and lowers cholesterol. There are two classifications of fiber: insoluble and soluble. Soluble fiber is found in oats, peas, rice, citrus, strawberries, and apple pulp and can reduce LDL (Low-density lipoprotein or "bad") cholesterol levels. Insoluble fiber is found in whole wheat breads, oatmeal, cabbage, beets, carrots, apple skin, and barley and can slow gastric emptying that leads to less eating.

Protein

Protein builds, maintains, and replaces the body's tissues. Muscles and organs are primarily made up of protein.

Carbohydrates

There are two different types of carbohydrates: simple (simple sugars) and complex (starches). The body breaks down carbohydrates into simple sugars, which are absorbed into the bloodstream. The pancreas releases insulin as the blood sugar rises. Insulin is what moves the sugar into the cells to make energy.

Fat

Fats are important to the diet as a source of energy and for the absorption of fat-soluble vitamins. Fats are identified in two ways: saturated and unsaturated. Saturated fats are usually animal fat and solid at room temperature. Unsaturated fats are usually vegetable fat and liquid at room temperature.

Cholesterol

Cholesterol is used to form cell membranes, some hormones and is needed for other body functions. It is a soft waxy substance found in every cell of the body and among the fats (lipids) in the bloodstream. Cholesterol cannot absorb in blood and is transported by lipoproteins. Two major lipoproteins are LDL (Low-density lipoprotein or "bad") and HDL (High-density lipoprotein or "good"). LDL is the major cholesterol carrier in the blood and can slowly build up on the walls of arteries. HDL carries cholesterol back to the liver where it can be passed by the body. Physical exercise can increase the HDL levels in the body.

VITAMINS

	Benefits	Sources
Vitamin A	keeps skin, hair, and nails healthy promotes cell growth prevents eye problems strengthens immune system lowers cholesterol levels helps protect against cancer	milk, eggs dark green vegetables orange vegetables orange fruits cereals
Vitamin B (B1, B2, B3, B5, B6, B9, B12)	involved with making red blood cells important for metabolic activity optimizes brain and mental alertness enhances circulation can reduce risk of heart disease regulates blood sugar protects against pollutants and toxins	whole grains fish and seafood poultry and meat milk, yogurt eggs leafy green vegetables beans, peas
Vitamin C	helps body absorb iron and calcium essential for healthy bones, teeth and blood vessels contributes to brain function helps body resist infection aids in wound healing strengthens blood vessels	tomatoes broccoli spinach, cabbage red berries red and green bell peppers citrus fruits, kiwi cantaloupe
Vitamin D	helps body absorb calcium, for healthy bones maintains body tissues (eyes, skin and liver) helps form red blood cells needed for cells to produce insulin: deficiency can lead to Type 1 Diabetes	body makes from sun exposure fish oils fortified milk and cereal liver egg yolks
Vitamin E	antioxidant that protects cells studies have shown protects against approximately 80 diseases reduces blood pressure promotes healthy skin and hair	whole grains leafy green vegetables wheat germ sardines egg yolks
Vitamin H	promotes healthy nerve tissue, bone marrow and sweat glands helps produce fatty acids aids in metabolizing energy, fats and proteins often recommended for hair and nail strengthening	tomatoes romaine lettuce, cabbage carrots, cucumbers almonds, walnuts eggs, milk onions, cauliflower raspberries, strawberries
Vitamin K	helps blood clotting	leafy green vegetables milk, yogurt, cheese broccoli, soybean oil

Eating

MINERALS

	Benefits	Sources
Calcium (Ca)	vital for strong bones and teeth	milk and dairy broccoli, fortified foods dark green leafy vegetables
Chlorine/ Chloride (Cl)	maintains fluid and electrolyte balance aids in digestion	salt, soy sauce milk, eggs, meat
Chromium (Cr)	required for release of energy from glucose (sugar)	vegetable oils liver, cheese, nuts whole grains
Copper (Cu)	necessary for absorption of iron supports formation of hemoglobin and several enzymes	meats water
Fluorine/ Floride (F)	involved with teeth and bone formation helps teeth resist decay	fluorinated drinking water tea seafood
Iodine (I)	part of thyroid hormones prevents goiter and infantile myxedema (birth defect)	iodized salt seafood kelp
Iron (Fe)	helps red blood cells carry oxygen	red meat, pork, poultry fish and shellfish lentils, beans, soy foods green leafy vegetables fortified foods
Magnesium (Mg)	helps muscles and nerves function keeps bones strong helps body create energy helps body make proteins regulates heart rhythm	whole grains, shrimp nuts and seeds green leafy vegetables potatoes, beans, tofu avocados, broccoli kiwi, bananas
Manganese (Mn)	facilitates cell processes	in many foods
Molybdenum (Mo)	facilitates cell processes	legumes organ meats
Phosphorus (P)	helps form healthy teeth and bones helps body make energy maintains acid-base balance every cell in the body contains and needs to function normally	dairy meat fish
Potassium (K)	helps muscles and nerves helps body maintain balance of water in blood and body tissues crucial for a healthy heart	broccoli, bananas potatoes (with skin) green leafy vegetables citrus fruits, dried fruits legumes (peas and lima beans)

MINERALS (CONT.)

	Benefits	Sources
Selenium (Se)	antioxidant, works with Vitamin E to protect body from oxidation	seafood, meats grains
Sodium (Na)	maintains fluid and electrolyte balance supports muscle contraction and nerve impulse transmissions	milk, bread meat salt, soy soy sauce
Sulfur (S)	important for protein structure necessary for energy metabolism, enzyme function and detoxification	meat eggs legumes
Zinc (Zn)	important for growth and sexual development helps immune systems promotes wound healing	red meat, poultry, nuts dairy products, soy foods oysters, seafood, dried beans whole grains, fortified foods

ORGANIC FOODS

All labeled organic foods must be made or produced by a set of production standards:

Non-livestock foods
- Grown without the use of conventional pesticides
- Grown without the use of artificial fertilizers
- Free of human or industrial waste contamination
- Processed without food additives or irradiation
- Free of artificial food additives

Livestock foods
- Reared without the use of antibiotics or growth hormones
- Generally fed a healthy diet
- Cannot be genetically modified in most countries

In the United States, processed organic foods (cereals, bread, etc.) must have at least 95% organic ingredients.

Organic food costs between 10-40% more than regularly processed food.

Studies have shown a higher nutrient content for some organic food compared to non-organic food, while other studies have shown no nutritional benefit over non-organic to organic food.

PERSONAL NOTES

Eating

Chapter 5

Sleeping

Sleep is as important to a baby as food. Many parents overlook this vital part of a child's development and rely on nature to take care of this by the phrase, "if he was tired, he would go to sleep...."

PERSONAL NOTES

SLEEP SCHEDULE

Every baby has different needs for sleep. The following table shows average sleep schedules for different ages.

Age	# of Naps	Night sleep	Total Sleep in 24 hours
0-1 month	4-6	-	16-20 hrs
2-3 months	3-4	5-8 hrs	15-17 hrs
4-6 months	3	8-12 hrs	15-16 hrs
7-8 months	2-3	10-12 hrs	14-16 hrs
8-12 months	2	10-12 hrs	14-15 hrs
12-18 months	1-2	10-12 hrs	12-14 hrs

SLEEP ADVICE

Many different methods that guarantee sleep are offered in books, magazines, and flyers. However, no method is necessarily easy. The list below has tips on promoting good sleep habits so Baby is happy when he or she is awake.

- Learn the cues Baby gives when tired. Some examples include yawning, rubbing eyes, gazing, slow blinks, and fussiness.
- Put a baby down when they give their sleepy cue, before they are too tired.
- If Baby consistently cries when put down flat in a bassinet or crib, they may have reflux and need to be inclined. Elevating the head of the mattress by placing something underneath or letting the baby sleep buckled in a car seat, bouncy seat, or swing can solve this. Discuss sleeping arrangements with Baby's pediatrician.
- Once a sleep schedule is established, protect it. Babies love and thrive on consistency.
- A fussy baby is usually sleepy, unless it is feeding time or they are hurt or sick.
- The crib should be a place to sleep, not play. Avoid putting crib toys and other stimulation where babies should be falling asleep. *(continued next page)*

Sleeping

- Avoid intentionally rocking to sleep. Rocking is soothing to babies, but does not let them learn to sleep in a normal non-rocking crib or bed.
- Baby's sleeping area should be as quiet as possible. This allows Baby to achieve a deeper sleep that is much more restful. If household noise is an issue, a white noise machine can be used on the lowest volume that drowns out other noises. Be sure to test the baby monitor to be sure Baby is detectable above the din.
- Baby's sleeping area should be darkened; this mutes visual stimulation and simulates a natural 'night' environment.
- Babies should wake up happy (cooing, talking) and not crying. If they wake up crying or fussy, they usually didn't get enough sleep unless it is past due for a feeding.
- A baby's sleep cycle is between 30-50 minutes. If Baby sleeps less than 30 minutes, they are not fully rested and should stay asleep. The more tired a baby is, the more difficult for them to fall and stay asleep.
- Since babies love consistency, try putting down with the same blanket or one stuffed animal (only if they are rolling over unassisted and are at least 9 months old).
- Bedtime should always be within a 30-minute time block every night. This establishes a healthy sleep routine. If Baby didn't take one or any of his naps and is extremely tired, it is best to put them down earlier. Great bedtimes for infants are between 6:30 and 8:30 pm.
- During night hours, limit interaction to simply feeding or changing the diaper. Avoid turning on the lights or talking to baby. This gives the infant the signal to wake up.

By three to four months of age:
- At this age, parents should start letting Baby fall asleep unassisted and start sleep training. Falling asleep without help is a learned behavior.
- Babies should be waking within the same 1-hour block of time every day. Some babies are early risers, while others tend to sleep in.
- Baby should be sleeping in a crib and preferably not in the parent's room. The transition to sleeping alone will become more difficult as the baby ages.
- If Baby awakes crying or prematurely, parents should wait 5-15 minutes to see if Baby will continue sleeping on their own.

Sleeping

SLEEP TRAINING

Sleep training, or letting an infant fall asleep unassisted, can be difficult for parents since it involves letting their baby cry to sleep. If parents stick to a consistent plan for 3-4 days, crying should be rare. Parents, remember to be patient!

NOTE: The optimum time to start letting an infant fall asleep unassisted by a caregiver is 3-4 months of age.

Some training guidelines:
- Be consistent. This is the most important. Without consistency, sleep training will fail because the infant never learns parent's intentions.
- Start training with naps first, as bedtime is always the most difficult.
- Establish a sleep routine to use EVERY time the infant is put to sleep. Sleep routines should be transferable to other locations and should be at least 5 steps long so the infant identifies the sleep routine. Sample routine sequences could be:
  - Change diaper, turn out light, rock for a minute, put down and close door
  - Change diaper, read a book, turn out light, close blinds, put down, give pacifier and leave room
- Once the infant has been put to bed, leave them alone (leave the room!) for at least 5 minutes, using a clock or timer. First time parents may find it very difficult to listen to their infant cry for 5 minutes straight.
- If Baby is still crying after 5 minutes, console and leave again for at least 5 minutes. Parents can choose to make this second "removal" for 10 minutes instead of 5 minutes, but be consistent every time!
- If they still are crying, console them and remove yourself again for at least 5 minutes. Parents can choose to make this third "removal" for 15 minutes, but be consistent.
- While training, never leave a baby crying for more than 15 minutes straight without consoling.
- If the infant stops crying for at least 20 seconds, and begins crying again the 5 minute time limit should restart when the crying resumes.
- Whichever method is chosen, the 5, 5, 5, 5-minute... or 5, 10, 15, 15-minute plan, it must be continued each time baby is put to sleep. *(continued next page)*

- Do not continue after an hour if Baby is still not asleep, unless it is bedtime. If after an hour, go and console Baby to sleep because they tend to be overtired and fight sleep harder; at that point they are not learning.
- Sleep training is harder for some infants than others. Be consistent and within a few days parents will be amazed at how much Baby has learned about self-comforting and falling asleep.
- Parents sometimes think they shouldn't leave a baby to comfort themselves, but it is a great tool for Baby to learn self-confidence and independence. The sound of a baby crying does not necessarily mean they are crying for mommy or daddy. They may cry because they are frustrated and want to sleep. Remember crying is the only way they can communicate.

SLEEPING THROUGH THE NIGHT

The age range for babies staying asleep for 8 hours (sleeping through the night) ranges from 2-9 months of age. Every baby is different and there are many books and articles on the subject.

Some common advice given:

- Night hours should be treated as sleep time at even the earliest age. Do not engage Baby during sleeping hours. Do not turn on the lights, talk, or sing to them during family "sleeping" hours.
- Once Baby is 3 months old, follow Baby's night sleep rhythm. If Baby goes for a certain time period, say 6 hours, without a night feeding for at least 3 consecutive nights do not let them breast feed or take a bottle if they wake up before that time. [Example: Bedtime is at 8pm. Baby starts waking for night feeding at 2am on Monday, Tuesday, and Wednesday night, but wakes up at 12:30 am on Thursday. Do not feed Baby until 2am, because Baby has already established that he or she can wait that long.]
- A *general* guideline for healthy babies: If Baby is more than 10 pounds, they should be able to go 6-8 hours between one feeding per 24 hours. If Baby is more than 14 pounds, they should be able to go 8-10 hours between one feeding per 24 hours. Remember, each baby is different.
- If Baby is not sleeping through the night at 5 months of age, try eliminating a night feeding if there is more than one, and just change diaper and console to sleep (do not talk or sing). Some babies require one night feeding until age 9 months. Elimination of a night feeding can be done by:
  - Realizing that they are feeding out of habit, not hunger
  - Increasing time between feedings by 15-20 minutes each night
  - Decreasing amount taken by 1 ounce or nursing 1 minute less each night
  - Never regress unless medically necessary

At 9 months of age, healthy babies no longer need a night feeding and are waking up due to a learned routine. This routine must be broken for Baby and parents to get a good night's sleep. Breaking this nightly ritual is very difficult because tired parents usually submit and feed the baby. Instead of feeding Baby reassure him briefly (without lights or loud talking) and leave, following the same 5, 5, 5-minute or 5, 10, 15-minute method introduced for naps before.

PERSONAL NOTES

Chapter 6

Baby Sign Language

Baby sign language is gaining popularity and is practiced more than ever. The chapter will give caregivers a brief overview on how to start signing and a few common baby signs using ASL, American Sign Language.

STARTING BABY SIGN LANGUAGE

- Begin signing as early as 5-6 months of age. It will take at least one month after caregivers begin signing for baby to begin signing back.
- Start with three basic signs. Do not do any other signs until baby masters these three.
- Every time caregivers speak the word, sign as well. Repetition, repetition, repetition.
- As many caregivers as possible should sign to baby for reinforcement.

AMERICAN SIGN LANGUAGE

Some common starting signs in the American Sign Language are in the following pages.

MOMMY   DADDY

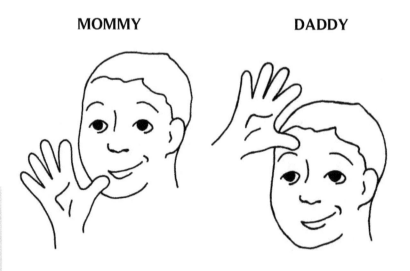

Baby Signs

MILK

SLEEP

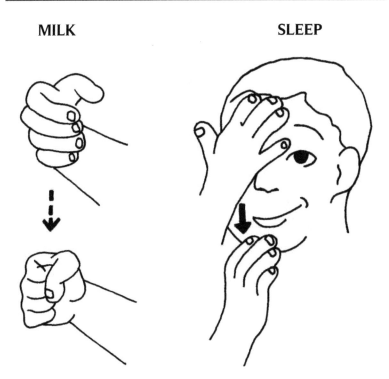

DRINK

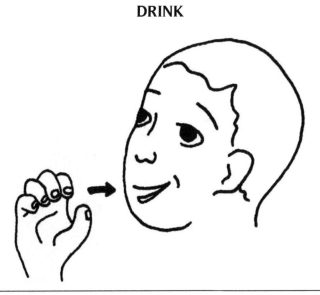

EAT

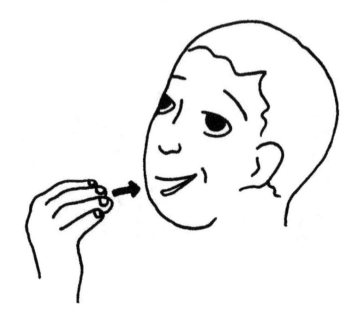

MORE

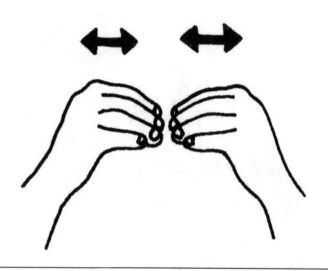

Baby Signs

DIAPER

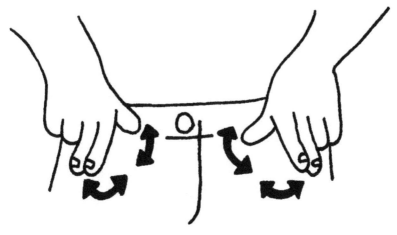

BOOK

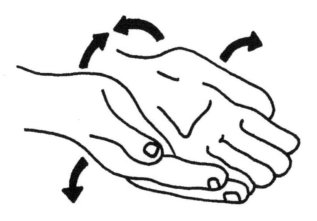

PLEASE

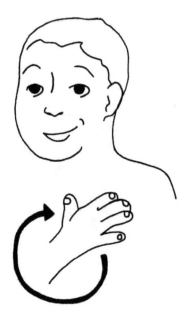

THANK YOU

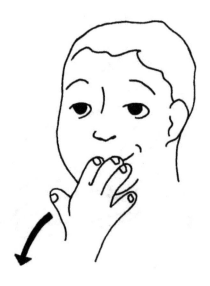

Baby Signs

Chapter 7

Health, Medicine & Illness

Unfortunately all infants will get sick; it is just a matter of how often and to what degree.

This chapter has information on a broad range of health issues including an immunization schedule with explanations, medicine dosages, serious illness symptoms, and common baby illnesses with home remedies.

Health

PERSONAL NOTES

Health

WELLNESS DOCTOR VISITS

Routine items a pediatrician should do during a wellness visit:
- Record height, weight, and head circumference
- Give scheduled immunizations
- Listen to heart and lung function
- Examine entire baby including eyes, ears, mouth, and genitalia
- Check development by asking parents questions on activities
- Review feeding, development, and safety items

A pediatrician will usually see a healthy baby for wellness visits on the following schedule: 2 or 3 days, 1 month, 2 months, 4 months, 6 months, 9 months, 12 months, 15 months, 18 months, 24 months, and 3 years of age.

IMMUNIZATION SCHEDULE

Below shows a common immunization schedule. Discuss with Baby's pediatrician for any variances or changes.

Age	Immunizations
Birth	Hep B
2 months	DTaP, Hep B, IPV, Hib, Prevnar, Rotavirus
4 months	DTaP, +/ Hep B, IPV, Hib, Prevnar, Rotavirus
6 months	DTaP, Hep B, IPV, Hib, Prevnar, Rotavirus
12 months	Hepatitis A, MMR, Varicella
15 months	Trihibit (or DTaP, Hib), Prevnar
18 months	Hepatitis A
4-6 years	DTaP, IPV, MMR, Varicella

Health

IMMUNIZATION TYPE SUMMARIES

Many immunizations today are combinations of different types of vaccines so a child need not be injected more than necessary. The following information outlines some common brand or verbal names of vaccines.

- DTaP – Provides protection against diphtheria, tetanus, and pertussis bacteria (whooping cough)
- Hepatitis A – Provides protection against Hepatitis A virus
- Hepatitis B (Hep B/HBV) – Provides protection against Hepatitis B virus
- Hib – Provides protection against Hib disease, Haemophilus influenza bacteria
- IPV - Provides protection against polio virus
- MMR – Provides protection against measles, mumps and rubella (German measles) viruses
- Pediarix– Combination of DTaP, IPV, and Hepatitis B virus
- Pentacel – Combination of DTaP, Hib, and IPV
- Prevnar – Provides protection against pneumococcal bacteria, PPV, PCV 7
- Rotateq/Rotarix – Provides protection against Rotavirus
- Trihibit – Combination of Tripedia (DTaP) & Hib
- Varicella – Provides protection against Varicella virus (Chicken pox)

DISEASES IMMUNIZATIONS PROTECT AGAINST

Disease	Spread By	Signs/Symptoms	Complications
Diphtheria (bacteria)	Air, Direct contact	Sore throat, mild fever, membrane in throat, swollen neck	Heart failure, paralysis, pneumonia, death
Hepatitis A (virus)	Personal contact; contaminated food or water	Fever, stomach pain, loss of appetite, fatigue, vomiting, jaundice, dark urine	Liver failure, death
Hepatitis B (virus)	Contact with blood or body fluids	Fever, headache, malaise, vomiting, arthritis	Chronic infection, cirrhosis, liver failure, liver cancer, death
Hib disease (bacteria)	Air, Direct contact	May be no symptoms unless bacteria enter blood	Meningitis, epiglotittis, pneumonia, arthritis, death
Influenza (virus)	Air, Direct contact	Fever, muscle pain, sore throat, cough	Pneumonia, Reye syndrome, myocarditis, death
Measles (virus)	Air, Direct contact	Rash, fever, cough, runny nose, pinkeye	Pneumonia, ear infections, encephalitis, seizures, death
Mumps (virus)	Air, Direct contact	Swollen throat, high fever, confusion	Meningitis, encephalitis, inflammation of testicles or ovaries, deafness
Pertussis (bacteria)	Air, Direct contact	Severe cough spells, runny nose, fever, vomiting with cough	Pneumonia, seizures, brain disorders, ear infection, death
Pneumococ-cal (bacteria)	Air, Direct contact	Pneumonia (fever, chills, cough, chest pain), ear infection	Bacteremia (blood infection), meningitis, death
Polio (virus)	Person to person	May be no symptoms, sore throat, fever, nausea	Paralysis, death
Rotavirus (virus)	Person to person, contaminated food or water	Diarrhea, vomiting, fever	Dehydration, electrolyte imbalance
Rubella (virus)	Air, Direct contact	Rash, fever, swollen glands	Encephalitis, arthritis/ arthralgia, bleeding, swollen testicles
Tetanus (bacteria)	Exposure through breaks in skin	Stiffness in neck, difficulty swallowing, rigid abdominal muscle, muscle spasms, fever, sweating, elevated blood pressure	Broken bones, breathing difficulty, death
Varicella (virus)	Air, Direct contact	Rash, fever	Bacterial infections, meningitis, encephalitis, pneumonia, death

*Information Source: Center of Disease Control, Parents' Guide to Immunizations 2008

BOWEL MOVEMENTS

Newborns and infants have an array of colors, consistencies, and frequencies in bowel movements. Routinely use diaper cream during the first few months of age while bowel movements are frequent to prevent diaper rash.

When to call the pediatrician:
- Blood or mucus present in stool (especially if darker red color)
- Bowel has a white color
- Black and tar looking (not including very first bowel movement)
- If exclusively breast feeding, no bowel movement in 7 days
- If exclusively formula feeding, no bowel movement in 2 days
- Consistency thicker than peanut butter if still on liquid only diet
- Green stool along with yellowish skin and/or eyes, if baby hasn't already been diagnosed with jaundice

If there is a questionable bowel movement, save and bring the diaper to the pediatrician for testing.

COLORS

Any colors ranging from yellow to yellow green are normal when exclusively breast feeding or formula feeding. Breast fed infant stools should be mustard colored, seedy and runny. Formula fed infant stools should be yellow to green and soft. Different colors and what they could mean are below.

Green
- Some infant formulas containing iron make stools change
- Foremilk/Hindmilk imbalance: Too much of the foremilk (less fatty) and not enough hind milk; sometimes caused by nursing too frequently or from only one breast
- Jaundice (liver not functioning correctly)
- Dairy Sensitivity, or cow's milk intolerance

Black
- Iron Supplements
- Intestinal bleeding, if stools are also tarry call doctor immediately

Dark Red or Raspberry
- Red food, if on solid foods (gelatin, juice, berries, etc)
- Small tears at anal opening from constipation
- Extreme diaper rash

Health

The first few days of an infant's bowel movements change from black, tarry to brown to yellowish. After the first week, the diaper usage remains fairly consistent for 3-4 weeks. At one month, the number of bowel movements, especially in breast fed infants, rapidly decreases.

Once solid foods are introduced, the bowel movements become more solid and change colors depending on the food given. Most often, certain foods cannot be digested (corn, pea hulls, etc.) and are found in the stools later.

SIGNS OF SERIOUS ILLNESS – WHEN TO CALL THE DOCTOR
If any of these symptoms are present, for the various ages, call the pediatrician for ***immediate*** *medical attention*.

NEWBORN – 2 MONTHS OF AGE
- Rectal temperature greater than 100.4° F
- Refuses to drink/eat for more than 4 hours
- Inconsolable crying for more than 2 hours
- Vomiting more than 6-8 hours or any blood
- More than 12 bowel movements in 24 hours
- Red belly button
- Change in breathing pattern
- Change in baby's color
- Seems floppy or limp

2 MONTHS – 12 MONTHS OF AGE
- Rectal temperature greater than 101° F for babies aged 2-6 months old
- Rectal temperature greater than 103° F for babies aged 6-12 months old
- Refusal to eat/drink at more than one feeding (over 6 hours)
- Extreme irritability
- Change in baby's color
- Inconsolable crying for more than 3-4 hours
- Extreme drowsiness
- Trouble breathing
- Bowel movements contain blood or mucus
- Vomiting more than 8 hours or any blood
- Diarrhea for more than 24 hours

(continued next page)

Health

- Dehydration symptoms: sunken eyes, sunken soft spot (on top of head), hands and feet that are cold and splotchy, fingers leave a white mark where skin was pressed for longer than 2 seconds, and no wet diaper for more than 8 hours – if more than two symptoms take to emergency room for intravenous fluid replenishment
- Pulls at one or both ears or has any discharge from ear

13 MONTHS – 36 MONTHS OF AGE

- Rectal temperature more than 103° F
- Trouble breathing
- Seizures or loss of consciousness
- Pulls at one or both ears or has any discharge from ear
- Stiff neck
- Refuses to eat/drink for 8 hours
- Vomiting for more than 12 hours or any blood
- Diarrhea for more than 72 hours (3 days)
- Discharge from ears or eyes
- Bowel movements contain blood or mucus
- Inability to walk normally (if able to walk)
- Blurred vision
- Loss of control of any body part (examples: leg, arm, feet, etc.) or sudden lethargy or inability to move
- Yellow hue to skin or eyes
- Pus from cut or scrape
- Dehydration symptoms: crying without tears, sunken eyes, sunken soft spot (on top of head), hands and feet that are cold and splotchy, fingers leave a white mark where skin was pressed for longer than 2 seconds, and no wet diaper for more than 8 hours – if more than two symptoms take to emergency room
- Complains of severe stomach pain, will not stop holding stomach, only stops crying if pressure is placed on stomach
- Cries when urinating

ACETAMINOPHEN DOSAGE (common brand Tylenol®)

Give no more than 5 times in a 24-hour period and no sooner than 4 hours apart. Before giving any medication to a child less than 2 years of age contact the pediatrician. Go by weight before age. Always use the dropper that comes with the medicine.

Age	Weight*	Drops 80 mg/ 0.8 ml	Elixir 160 mg/ 5 ml
0 to 3 months *ask doctor before	6 to 11 lbs. (2.7 to 5 kg)	40 mg: 1/2 dropper Infant Concentrated Drops	—
4 to 11 months	12 to 17 lbs. (5.5 to 7.7 kg)	80 mg: 1 dropper Infant Concentrated Drops	1/2 tsp. Children's Liquid
1 to 2 years	18 to 23 lbs. (8.2 - 10.4 kg)	120 mg:1 1/2 droppers Infant Concentrated Drops	3/4 tsp. Children's Liquid
2 to 3 years	24 to 35 lbs. (8.2 - 10.4 kg)	160 mg: 2 droppers Infant Concentrated Drops	1 tsp. Children's Liquid

IBUPROFEN (common brand Advil® or Motrin®)

Give no more than 5 times in a 24-hour period and no sooner than every 6 hours. Before giving any medication to a child less than 2 years of age contact the pediatrician. Go by weight before age. Always use the dropper that comes with the medicine.

Age	Weight*	Drops 50 mg/ 1.25 ml	Suspension 100 mg/ 5 ml
6 to 12 months	12 to 17 lbs. (5.5 to 7.7 kg)	1.25 ml: 1 dropper Infant Concentrated Drops	-
1 to 2 years	18 to 23 lbs. (8.2 - 10.4 kg)	1.875 ml: 1 1/2 droppers Infant Concentrated Drops	-
2 to 3 years	24 to 35 lbs. (8.2 - 10.4 kg)	2.5 ml: 2 droppers Infant Concentrated Drops	1 tsp. Children's Suspension

Health

UNIT CONVERSIONS

All unit conversions have been rounded for simplicity.

1 milliliter (ml) = 1/5 US teaspoon (US tsp)
1 US tsp = 5 ml = 1/3 US tablespoon
1 US Tbsp = 3 US tsp = 1/16 Cup
1 US fluid ounce (US fl oz) = 30 ml
1 UK fluid ounce (UK fl oz) = 28 ml
1 dry ounce (oz) = 2 Tbsp = 6 tsp = 1/8 Cup = 28 grams (g)

REDUCING SICKNESS

Some sicknesses cannot be avoided, but reducing the risk to Baby can be done by:

1.) Washing hands before handling a baby and after diaper changes
2.) Disinfecting bottles, toys, and teethers frequently (see next section on disinfecting)
3.) Avoiding contact with other sick people when possible
4.) Avoiding physical contact with public items as much as possible, especially at medical care facilities
5.) Administering flu shot if infant is over 6 months of age
6.) Clothing infants properly, not too warm or too cold

NOTE: If a breast feeding mother gets sick, she can still nurse her infant, unless her doctor explicitly states otherwise.

Health

DISINFECTING

Disinfecting by steam or boiling is preferred because no chemicals are involved; however, common household bleach can also be used. Always wash items (with soapy water and rinse) before disinfecting.

BOILING: Item must be fully submerged and boiled for at least 5 minutes to disinfect thoroughly.

STEAM: Item must be steamed for at least 3 minutes. Steam can easily burn because of the high temperature – be careful!

BLEACH: Regular household bleach can be diluted to different concentrations to disinfect. After surface or item has been soaked or wiped with a bleach concentration, be sure to rinse or wipe with water thoroughly. The table below shows different bleach concentrations for different household uses. *Be sure surface is bleach safe (it will permanently discolor most fabrics, carpets, upholstery, etc.)*

Item Disinfecting	Part Household Bleach	Part Water	Ratio	Soak Time
Bottles, Teething Rings, Cups, Nipples, Pacifiers	1 tablespoon	1 gallon	1:256	2 minutes
Non-mouthed Plastic Toys, Highchairs, Bleach Safe Floors, Sponges, Appliances, General Disinfecting	3/4 cup	1 gallon	1:12	5 minutes
Laundry, Cloth Diapers	3/4 cup	regular wash load	-	wash cycle
	1 1/4 cup	extra large wash load	-	wash cycle

Health

COMMON BABY ILLNESSES AND DISCOMFORTS

No book, chart or table can replace a pediatrician, and if at any time something isn't right – call the pediatrician or nurse.

Typical viruses can last for 7-10 days. If Baby has been sick or has had any uncommon behaviors for more than that time, call the pediatrician promptly because something serious may be wrong.

Antibiotics prescribed by a pediatrician only treat bacterial infections, not viral infections.

COLD OR INFLUENZA

The common cold and influenza (flu) are both respiratory illnesses but are caused by different viruses. The two illnesses share similar symptoms such as fever, body aches, extreme tiredness, and dry cough. Reaction to the flu is generally more severe than the common cold. Cold infections usually include runny nose and sore throat but do not result in serious health problems such as pneumonia, bacterial infections, or hospitalization.

Because the common cold and influenza viruses share many symptoms, it can be difficult (or even impossible) to tell the difference between them based on symptoms alone.

Babies can be vaccinated for seasonal influenza starting at 6 months of age.

Health

COLIC

Colic is a term describing a baby who is fussy and cries for up to 3 hours a day. Colic affects some babies from a few weeks old until 4 months of age. The causes for colic are unknown. Consult Baby's pediatrician to rule out any serious problems or health concerns.

Babies cry because it is the only form of communication and they are trying to tell you they are:
- Hungry
- Tired
- Need to pass gas
- In pain
- Wanting to cuddle or have contact (some babies are very sensitive to this)
- Too hot or too cold (feel Baby's head for hot, hands/feet for cold)
- Drank milk too quickly from a bottle (try a smaller nipple)
- Itch (from clothing, tags, hair, etc.)

Try the following to soothe Baby:
- Hold and/or walk Baby
- Sing to Baby
- Change positions (including leg pumping or sitting upright)
- Take a car or stroller ride
- Put in a baby swing
- Continuous noise or vibration (either from a sound machine, washer, static, etc)
- Place slight pressure on tummy or try burping
- Give Baby a bath

Some infants can have food intolerances and can exhibit colic-like symptoms. Breast fed infants can have food intolerances from foods passed through from the mother's diet. See Food Intolerance section.

Health

CONSTIPATION

An infant has constipation when their bowel movements are firm, dry, and/or pebbly. It is the consistency that determines constipation, not the frequency or the amount of effort exerted. The causes of constipation are: 1) insufficient fluids, 2) new foods, 3) low fiber, 4) different types of formula, and 5) medications. It is rare for a breast fed infant to get constipation.

When to call the doctor:
- Cries while straining
- Not gaining weight
- Frequent constipation
- Blood in stool
- If exclusively breast feeding, no bowel movement in 7 days
- If exclusively formula feeding, no bowel movement in 2 days

What to do for constipation at different ages is below.

Birth to 6 months of age:
1.) If formula fed, check preparation accuracy.
2.) Add 1 oz. of boiled then cooled water to formula preparation ONCE a day or offer 1 oz. of electrolyte solution to breast fed infants.

6 months of age and over:
1.) Offer diluted fruit juice (half water), no more than 4-6 oz.
2.) Offer mixed grain cereal (for fiber).
3.) Increase fruits and vegetables offered.
4.) Try to increase baby's activity level.
5.) Cut down on milk food products (cheese, yogurt, custard).

Health

DIAPER RASH

Beyond using topical over-the-counter baby diaper rash ointment, try:

1.) Frequent diaper changes
2.) After bowel movements, give short bath and air or pat bottom dry
3.) Be sure diaper area is completely dry before applying an antifungal cream or ointment and then a diaper cream to protect from future moisture
4.) Let baby go diaper-less as much as possible

Prevention: Application of diaper cream routinely until stools are much less frequent, especially to breast fed infants who have more frequent stools that can cause rashes easily, can cut down on breakouts.

If rash lasts longer than 3-4 days or develops blisters, call the pediatrician.

Yeast Infections

Boys and girls can develop yeast infections in their diaper area. The rash doesn't respond to usual over-the-counter diaper creams. It requires an antifungal cream. The skin is a bright red and very well defined with slightly raised borders; it could also look scaly.

Babies are more susceptible to yeast infections when they are on an antibiotic or after they have had thrush (yeast infection of the mouth). If Baby needs antibiotics and is more than 6 months old, feeding them yogurt or using pediatric probiotics may prevent this infection. See Probiotics section.

Health

DIARRHEA

Minor stomach viruses or food intolerance causes many cases of diarrhea. If Baby is trying new foods, the new one may be the culprit; discontinue and see if stools resume to normal. If it is a stomach bug, pediatricians usually give no medical treatment and just let it run its course. Diarrhea by itself isn't an emergency unless accompanied by other symptoms.

 When to call the doctor:
- Diarrhea accompanied by a fever
- Any dehydration symptoms develop - no wet diaper for more than 6-8 hours, no tears, hands/feet cold and clammy, dry mouth, fingers leave a white mark where skin was pressed for longer than 2 seconds, sunken soft spot (on top of head), etc.
- Diarrhea continues for a longer period of time than stated in signs of serious sickness section for given age

Things to do:
1.) Replenish lost fluids by offering fluids more frequently. Do not give water or dilute formula for infants less than 6 months of age. Never give babies or toddlers that have diarrhea only water or diluted electrolyte solution since they need more sugar and electrolytes.
2.) Use diaper cream to avoid rashes.
3.) If over the age of 6 months, dilute breast milk or formula with half electrolyte fluid.
   If over 12 months of age, give straight electrolyte solution in a sippy cup or bottle.
4.) If eating solid foods, do not feed any vegetables or fruits that start with the letter "p" (peas, prunes, pears, etc.).

Health

EAR INFECTION

The only treatment for ear infections is prescribed antibiotics by a pediatrician. About half of ear infections resolve themselves without treatment. If it is minor and only causing minimal discomfort, wait a few days because it is beneficial to minimize the number of times a child takes antibiotics. Ear infections need to be medically treated if they cause disinterest in eating or Baby's temperature rises to above 101.5° F (any age) for 2 consecutive days.

Factors that can increase the risk of ear infections are:
* Exposure to cigarette smoke
* Drinking from a horizontal position (allows fluid to go into ears)
* Formula fed instead of breast fed
* Attending daycare or nurseries when less than 12 months of age
* Use of a pacifier
* Frequent spitting

FEVER

A natural way to relieve a child's fever is to give them a lukewarm bath - never with cold water. Do not overdress an infant as this can increase the fever. Make sure baby is drinking enough fluids. If Baby will not stay in a bath, undress and wrap with towels soaked in warm water.

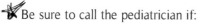 Be sure to call the pediatrician if:
* A fever does not lower at all within one hour of administering acetaminophen or ibuprofen
* Rectal temperature greater than:
  * 100.4° F for babies less than 2 months of age
  * 101° F for babies aged 2-6 months of age
  * 103° F for babies aged 6-12 months of age

Never give acetaminophen to babies 2 months of age or younger. Ibuprofen should not be administered before 6 months of age.

Rectal and oral temperatures are the only reliable way of monitoring a fever. Measuring by the forehead or armpit are reasonable alternatives but there is no official conversion to actual rectal temperature to serve as a good estimate. Ear thermometers are unreliable because of earwax buildup and possible ear infections.

Health

FOOD INTOLERANCE

Some infants can have sensitivity, intolerance, or an allergy to certain food(s). Anyone can have an intolerance or allergy to anything, however, the seven most common food intolerances (making up approximately 90% of all) are: dairy, wheat, soy, tree nuts, peanuts, shellfish, and egg whites. These are listed in nutritional information section of food labels. The most common food intolerance for infants is dairy (or cow's milk protein) and most will outgrow by 5-18 months of age.

Diagnosing is sometimes difficult because: 1) babies cry for other reasons, 2) food in mother's diet takes 4-8 hours to be transferred to breast milk, 3) the food in mother's diet can linger in breast milk production for up to 2 weeks, and 4) symptoms can show up minutes or hours after eating the food (or affected breast milk).

Common symptoms of food intolerance are:
- Crying or inconsolability 5 minutes to 2 hours after eating
- Vomiting
- Diarrhea (with or without mucus)
- Hives
- Blood in stools
- Difficulty breathing or wheezing
- Stomach cramping
- Swelling or itching (especially of lips, tongue or mouth)
- Dry, scaly, or red skin patches

Some facts on food intolerance:
- Varies in severity
- Dose related (small portions may be acceptable)
- Symptoms can change with age
- Should not interfere with child's growth
- If allergic to a particular food, could also be allergic to other foods in that group
- Cow's milk intolerance can cause green stools

If food intolerance is suspected in breast fed infants, try:
- A maternal food record (with items eaten, time, and infant symptoms)
- Mother starts an elimination diet

Because proper nutrition is crucial to an infant's development, consult the pediatrician if food intolerance is suspected.

Health

GAS & BURPING

Most infants, especially newborns under 13 weeks of age, have gas because of their immature digestive system. Infants tend to swallow excess air when feeding or screaming which causes extreme discomfort. Gas discomfort will decrease with age as Baby gets better at eating and their digestive system develops.

Things that minimize gas:
- Breast feeding with proper seal around nipple
- Feeding in an upright position (at least 45 degree incline)
- Smaller feedings
- Proper bottle nipple size (if too big, baby will eat too fast and if too small, baby will gulp air)
- Not over stimulating baby (by causing stress)

Symptoms of gas and the need to be burped:
- Stops in the middle of feeding and cries – refuses to drink remainder
- Arched back
- Squirm or grimace when laid down

Things crucial to expelling gas while burping:
- Holding baby upright
- Putting slight pressure on tummy
- Gently patting or rubbing back

NASAL CONGESTION

Nasal congestion may sound worse than it is; babies will breathe deeper/wheeze/sneeze if they need help or are bothered by the congestion. Treatment is only necessary if congestion is interfering with eating and/or sleeping. Unfortunately, the only relief that pediatricians recommend is:
- Cool-mist humidifier in the immediate area where the child plays and sleeps
- Nasal aspiration (or bulb plunger) as necessary
- Saline drops (just a couple) in nostrils to help loosen mucus
- Raise head of bed by putting rolled blanket under mattress or from floor, do not use a pillow inside crib sleeping area unless greater than 12 months old

Health

REFLUX

Reflux is another term for GER, Gastro Esophageal Reflux, and is the backward flow of stomach contents up into the throat. When GER causes complications or long-term problems, it is referred to as GERD, or Gastro Esophageal Reflux Disease.

Many infants have some symptoms of reflux, but very few have GERD causing serious health concerns. Some symptoms of reflux, GER, and GERD are:
- Constant or sudden crying or colic-like symptoms
- Poor sleep habits, typically with frequent waking
- Arching their necks and back during or after eating
- Spitting-up or vomiting
- Wet burp or frequent hiccups
- Frequent ear infections or sinus congestion
- Refusing food or accepting only a few bites despite being hungry
- Requiring constant small meals or liquid
- Food/oral aversions
- Excessive drooling
- Running nose, sinus infections
- Swallowing problems, gagging, choking
- Hoarse voice
- Frequent red, sore throat without infection
- Sleep apnea
- Respiratory problems—pneumonia, bronchitis, wheezing, asthma, night-time cough, aspiration
- Gagging themselves
- Poor weight gain, weight loss, or anemia
- Neck arching (Sandifer's Syndrome)
- Bad breath

Some things to reduce reflux in infants:
- Smaller and more frequent feedings
- Keep Baby at an inclined position during feeding, 30 minutes after feeding, and while sleeping (around a 30 degree incline is best)
- Keep clothes loose around stomach

Be sure to discuss any reflux symptoms with the pediatrician because if left untreated, symptoms may worsen.

TEETHING

Teething is the term used for emerging teeth, which can happen between 3 and 36 months of age. It is normal for some infants to get many teeth at an early age or not to get any for a while. It is not abnormal for infants not to have teeth at 12 months of age.

The only known associations with teething are drooling, fussiness, chewing, and an increase in the looseness of stools. Don't blame symptoms on teething until the tooth can be seen.

While infants are teething (usually only a few days for each tooth), they tend to drool excessively and want to chew on things.

Teething for some infants can be very painful and they may be very irritable and cranky. Teething can cause a slight fever, but if a true fever (values stated in Fever section) or diarrhea develops contact the pediatrician.

Some things to do:
- Let Baby chew on cool (not frozen) cloths, teething rings, or other large items they can hold on to and not choke. Frozen solid objects may bruise gums causing more discomfort.
- Use topical teething gel on gums to reduce pain no more than what label states. The first time Baby uses teething gel watch closely as some babies are allergic.
- Wipe excess drool from face to prevent a rash from developing.
- Give acetaminophen if pain seems to interrupt eating or sleeping.
- Do not use teething tablets because they are unproven and contain Belladonna (known to cause seizures in epileptic infants).

Once an infant has teeth, those teeth must be cleaned at least once a day by wiping a wet cloth across them. Do not use toothpaste until they are old enough to spit it out, usually by 2-3 years of age.

Health

VOMITING

Most toddlers and infants vomit from gastroenteritis, or stomach flu, and it is often accompanied by diarrhea and nausea. Stay calm and give plenty of fluids; dehydration can be very serious.

When to call the pediatrician:
- Vomit has blood or looks like it has coffee grounds (dried blood)
- Vomiting with a fever
- Vomiting continues after child has been given electrolyte fluid for 24 hours
- Vomiting resumes when trying to resume normal diet
- Projectile vomiting under 18 months of age
- Vomiting starts immediately after a head injury
- Vomit has green or yellowish-green color
- Belly feels bloated, hard, and/or is painful between vomiting episodes
- If under 1 month of age and vomits entire feeding
- If under 6 months of age, vomiting continues for more than 8 hours
- Any dehydration symptoms develop - no wet diaper for more than 6-8 hours, no tears, hands/feet cold and clammy, dry mouth, fingers leave a white mark where skin was pressed for longer than 2 seconds, sunken soft spot (on top of head), etc.

Some things to do for different ages are below.

Birth to 6 months of age:
1.) Do not give plain water unless instructed by the pediatrician.
2.) Offer 1/2 ounce of electrolyte solution every 20 minutes with oral syringe or bottle; do not give infant more electrolyte solution than they would normally eat (can cause upset stomach).
3.) Gradually offer more electrolyte solution every time offered until they are receiving entire feeding of electrolyte solution (instead of breast milk or formula).
4.) *IF formula fed and goes 4 hours without vomiting*, reintroduce formula slowly by giving ½ formula and ½ electrolyte solution for one feeding. If baby does not vomit, resume normal feeding regime.

(#4 continued next page)

Health

IF breast fed and goes 4 hours without vomiting, start breast feeding for 5-10 minutes every 2 hours and gradually increase duration of feeding and time between feedings.

6 months to 12 months of age:
1.) Follow above steps, but introduce bland solid foods (crackers, bananas, cereal) after 8 hours of no vomiting and continue normal diet after 24 hours of no vomiting.

12 months of age and above:
1.) Give clear liquids every 15 minutes (milk and milk products should be avoided).
2.) After 8 hours of no vomiting, introduce bland foods (crackers, bananas, cereal, mashed potatoes, rice, toast, mild soup, etc). Do not force child to eat.
3.) After 24 hours of no vomiting, continue regular diet with exception of milk and milk products. Resume milk products after 48 hours of no vomiting.

Health

PROBIOTICS

Probiotics can be used to help offset side effects from antibiotics (cramping, gas, diaper rash, or diarrhea) and lactose intolerance (enzyme deficiency for proper digestion of milk products).

Probiotics are live microorganisms that are similar to those found in the human digestive system, and more commonly known as "good bacteria". They are found in some foods such as yogurt, but are also sold as dietary supplements.

A person's "good bacteria" is vital to proper development of their immune system, for protection against other microorganisms that could cause disease, and to the digestion and absorption of food and nutrients. Every person's mix of bacteria differs but can be thrown off balance in the following ways:
- Using antibiotics
- Unfriendly microorganisms, such as yeast, fungi and parasites

Some research found that some probiotic formulations have helped with the following conditions:
- Diarrhea
- Urinary tract infections
- Irritable bowel syndrome (IBS)
- Atopic dermatitis (eczema) in children
- Intestinal infection durations from *Clostridium difficile* bacteria

Everyone can react differently to probiotic use*. **Always consult a pediatrician before starting a supplement of any kind. If a child is already taking probiotics be sure to inform the pediatrician.***

Health

Chapter 8

Safety & First Aid

The first aid portion of this chapter hopefully will never be used. Please read it carefully to be prepared for an emergency if one were to happen. Keep this book, or another first aid guide, handy and accessible for all caregivers at all times.

Always call 911 if the emergency is overwhelming or life threatening.

Never put yourself in danger to help someone else. You will not be able to help them if you are injured yourself.

Refer to the back pages for baby sitter checklist and important emergency phone numbers.

PERSONAL NOTES

SIDS

Doctors do not know the causes of Sudden Infant Death Syndrome (SIDS), but have identified certain risk factors from case studies. In a typical SIDS case, parents find their infant not breathing in his or her crib.

Babies that are at a higher risk for SIDS are: low weight or preterm, between one and six months of age, male, African American or Native American ethnicity, born in fall or winter months, and born to mothers that smoke or use illegal drugs.

Parents can reduce the risk of SIDS by the following:
- Pregnant mothers should avoid smoking and using illegal drugs
- Put Baby to sleep on their backs; even if they like sleeping on their stomachs
- Firm crib mattress
- Keep Baby's crib or bassinet in parent's room until 6 months of age
- Do not let Baby sleep in parent's bed or fall asleep with baby on a couch or chair
- Do not over clothe Baby while sleeping by dressing too warm
- Do not make room too warm (should be comfortable to adult)
- Avoid exposure to tobacco smoke
- Breast feed
- Try to limit or avoid contact with people who have respiratory infections
- Offer a pacifier

If Baby ever does the following, **call 911**:
- Goes limp
- Turns blue
- Periods of not breathing
- Gags excessively or stops breathing after spitting up

CHILD PROOFING

Child proofing a home does not mean that a child can be left unattended. It will help prevent first-aid issues and also give parents a little peace of mind. Many products are marketed that offer safety protection for different areas of the home. When child proofing a home, remember these areas:

- Stairs, balconies and banisters
- Cabinets
- Drawers
- Door stops (tips can come off and are a choking hazard)
- Lazy Susan turntables
- Stove
- Fireplace including mantle
- Electrical outlets
- Electrical cords
- Decorative items on top of furniture (picture frames, figurines)
- Window blind/shade cords
- Furniture that could tip when pulled or climbed, especially TV stands
- Coffee and side table corners and drawers/cabinets
- Toilets
- Door hinges (pinch fingers)
- Bi-fold closet doors (pinch fingers)
- Lamp cords
- Table cloths
- Upstairs windows that are routinely open (screens can tear)
- Kitchen knives need to be in a locked drawer/cabinet
- Chemicals, cleaning products, and poisonous items
- Medicines
- Poisonous plants, indoor and outdoor
- Space heaters should be marked by independent laboratory (such as UL, ETA, CSA listed), not closer than 3 feet to anything that can burn (fabric, wood, plastic, etc.), should not be used when not in the room or sleeping
- Swimming pools and outdoor water fountains, ponds, etc.

HOUSE SAFETY

Items to make a safer home for infants and children.
- Kitchen fire extinguisher
- Carbon monoxide detector/Smoke alarms in hallways and living spaces, at least one per level of a home
- First-aid kit properly stocked
- Water heater thermostat turned down to 120° F or below
- Fire escape plans for children's rooms
- Emergency phone numbers posted by phone

OUT & ABOUT SAFETY

Many accidents can be prevented. Remember these items when taking baby places.
- Always have baby in car seat properly sized and installed when in a vehicle. A parked vehicle is a potential target for an accident.
- Always use the provided straps on shopping carts to keep infants and toddlers safe. They can climb/fall out in an instant.
- Never place a baby in direct sunlight. If going outdoors, **always** use sunscreen of SPF 30 or higher. *NOTE:* Sunscreen labels state never to use on babies less than 6 months because they should not be in the sun at all.

EMERGENCY PREPAREDNESS

It is important to make a family plan for any type of emergency – natural or human (examples: tornadoes, hurricanes, earthquakes, terrorist attacks, etc.). The plan should include at a minimum:
- Lists of important phone numbers, addresses, and email addresses (email may work if cell phones do not)
- An out of town contact plus a location away from home where all family members can report to if separated or home is unavailable
- Keep at least a half tank of fuel in vehicle at all times (gas pumps do not work without electricity)
- Supply/restock a disaster supply kit every 6 months
- Know how to turn off home's electricity, water, and gas
- If evacuation is possible for the area, have essentials packed
- A "what if" plan that considers things that may not be available in an emergency (roadways blocked, cell phones not working, mass transit not available, power outage, etc.)
- Understand disaster plans of schools, caregivers, and local authorities *(continued next page)*

A disaster supply kit should have enough equipment to withstand an emergency for **at least three days**. If possible, store kit in a sealed container(s) indoors. A list should contain items that cannot be assembled beforehand (medicines, clothing, etc.).

Basics for family:

- First aid kit
- Flashlight and candles
- Battery operated radio
- Extra batteries for flashlights and radio
- Disposable gloves, sealable bucket, and bleach for disinfecting
- Kitchen items: can opener, knife, sugar, salt, disposable utensils, plates, cups, and plastic wrap
- Soap and/or hand sanitizer
- Heavy duty plastic bags with ties for sanitation
- Extra set of keys and identification
- Cash, coins, and copies of credit cards
- Copies of medical prescriptions
- Area map, compass, and shovel
- Shampoo, toothpaste, sunscreen, comb, toilet paper, and feminine supplies
- Matches in waterproof container
- Pet supplies: food, extra water, leash, and bedding

The bare basics for *each* family member:

- 1 gallon of drinking water per day
- 3 gallons of non-drinking water per day
- Three meals per day (should not need to be cooked)
- Blankets and coats if necessary
- Bedding, washcloth, and towel
- Disposable poncho or rain gear
- Medications
- Toothbrush
- Extra set of clothing and shoes
- Infants/toddlers: canned formula if needed, disposable diapers, bags for soiled diapers, baby food, special bedding, evaporated milk if over 12 months old, pacifier, toys, books, and teething ring if needed

FIRST AID

If at any time you feel as though you are not in control of a situation or it is life threatening, call 911 or your doctor immediately.

Never put yourself in danger to help someone else. You will not be able to help them if you are injured yourself.

BONE FRACTURES

Bone fractures always require medical attention. If the bone fracture or break is a result of a major trauma or fall, call 911.

If the following is also present, call 911:

- If Baby is unresponsive or not breathing, start CPR until help arrives
- Massive bleeding
- Gentle pressure causes pain
- Limb or joint looks deformed
- Bone fracture is in the head, neck, back, hip, pelvis, or upper leg
- Extremity of injured part (finger or toe) is numb or bluish
- Bone has pierced the skin

Things to do while waiting for medical attention:

1.) Keep area still; don't try to splint unless you are trained to do so, don't try to move or re-align the bone.
2.) Stop any bleeding by applying direct pressure with a sterile gauze or clean cloth.
3.) Apply ice packs to area to limit swelling; do not put ice directly on skin – wrap in towel or cloth.
4.) Treat shock if present; if Baby looks pale, dizzy, or is breathing fast - lie down (or hold as still as possible) and elevate legs, if possible.

BURNS or SCALDING

Children are inquisitive and often get burned from hot water, stoves, light bulbs, and heaters. The three types of burns, first, second, and third degree, have differing treatments. Any first degree burn that is more than 3 inches, any second degree, or any third degree burn needs to be seen by the pediatrician.

MINOR BURN TREATMENT

If burn is red, has pain and/or swelling with blisters, and less than 2 inches in diameter, treat as follows:

1.) Cool the burn with cool running water, or cool compress, for at least 5 minutes. Do not use ice.
2.) Apply aloe-vera gel or burn cream if over 6 months of age. Do not use butter or petroleum based ointments. Be careful not to break any blisters.
3.) Loosely cover burn with sterile gauze or bandage. Do not use cotton balls or pads as they can stick to burn.
4.) Once HEALED use sunscreen on scar for a year to minimize discoloration.

MAJOR BURN TREATMENT

If burn is greater than 3 inches in diameter and/or is black, white, and painless, **always call 911 or seek IMMEDIATE medical attention**. Follow these steps until help arrives:

1.) Do not remove burnt clothing, but do remove from source of heat, if safely possible.
2.) Do NOT submerge in water! This can cause shock.
3.) If Baby is not moving, coughing or breathing, begin CPR.
4.) Elevate burned parts above heart level if possible.
5.) Cover the area of the burn with cool moist sterile bandage or clean moist cloth or towel.

First Degree Burn – Only first layer of skin is burned; will be red and have pain or burning. Treat as a MINOR burn unless it is more than 3 inches in diameter or involves a major joint, face, buttocks, or groin.

Second Degree Burn – The first and second layer of skin is burned; will be accompanied by blisters and/or red blotchy skin with severe pain and swelling. Treat as a MINOR burn if less than 2 inches in diameter. Treat as a MAJOR burn if more than 2 inches in diameter and/or includes a major joint, the hands, feet, face, buttocks or groin.

Third Degree Burn – All layers of the skin are burned. May appear black, charred dry and white and are painless. Treat as a MAJOR burn. _ALWAYS_ _seek immediate medical attention._

CHOKING

Many babies when trying new foods will experience an episode of choking. The risk of choking can be reduced if the child is always seated and supervised when eating.

Most of the time a gentle pat on the back or a finger swipe into their mouth clears it. However, if Baby is NOT coughing, stops breathing, and starts turning red or blue immediately perform the emergency choking steps below. **Basic steps: give 5 back blows and 5 chest compressions, repeat until help arrives.** Follow the instructions below for the different ages.

CHOKING (12 months old and younger)
Steps:
1.) If you are with someone, have him or her call 911.
2.) Sit down with Baby in lap face down with one arm under Baby's chest.
3.) With other hand gently but firmly give 5 back blows to the middle of the back.

If that doesn't work:

4.) Turn Baby over, to face upwards, in the same position (resting on your forearm).
5.) Give Baby five quick chest compressions with two fingers at base of breastbone.
6.) If Baby still isn't breathing, call 911 if you are by yourself.
7.) Repeat five back blows and 5 chest compressions until medical help arrives.
8.) If airway becomes open and Baby doesn't start coughing or breathing on own, start CPR immediately.

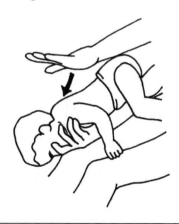

CHOKING (13 months to 3 years old)

Treatment of choking emergencies for toddlers over 12 months old is the same as an adult. **Two basic elements: 5 back blows and 5 abdominal thrusts (Heimlich maneuver).**

Steps:
1.) If you are with someone, have him or her call 911.
2.) Lay toddler on floor face down.
3.) Deliver five back blows with the heel of your hand between their shoulder blades.
4.) Give five abdominal thrusts:
   a. Stand behind toddler or have them seated on your lap facing away from you.
   b. Wrap your arms around their waist and lean them forward a little.
   c. Make a fist with one hand and wrap your other hand around it.
   d. Quickly press up into the abdomen a couple finger widths below the chest bone five times; this step should be as though you are quickly trying to lift the toddler up.
5.) If the airway is still blocked, and you are alone call 911. Repeat the five back blows to five abdominal thrusts until help arrives.
6.) If the airway becomes open and the toddler doesn't start coughing or breathing, proceed to CPR.

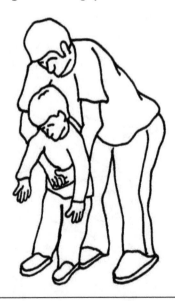

CPR (CARDIOPULMONARY RESUSCITATION)

Cardiopulmonary resuscitation, CPR, is used in emergencies when a person's heart and/or breathing have stopped. It involves two elements: **mouth-to-mouth breathing and chest compressions**.

When the heart stops, it only takes a few minutes to cause brain damage and 8-10 minutes for death. CPR can keep oxygenated blood circulating until more medical attention can be given. This is crucial in saving your baby's life. **Parents should take a certified and accredited class on first aid and CPR.**

Children are almost always in respiratory failure unlike adults who are almost always in cardiac emergencies. In general, airway and breathing is more important for children and circulation more important for adults.

The steps outlined in the following pages were taken from the American Heart Association 2005 guidelines for CPR. If you have not been trained in CPR, eliminate the breathing section and focus on the airway and circulation (chest compressions).

(continued next pages)

CPR FOR INFANTS (less than 12 months old)

Assess the situation. Stroke the baby, do not shake, and wait for a response.

If there is no response:

1.) Either have someone call 911 or if you are by yourself, give CPR for 2 minutes before calling for help.

2.) BEGIN the ABC's of CPR: Airway, Breathing and Circulation

AIRWAY (clearing airway)

1.) Place Baby face up on a firm, flat surface (table or floor is fine).

2.) Tip the head back gently by lifting the chin with one hand and pressing down on the forehead with the other.

3.) Put ear next to Baby's mouth and listen and look for breathing for no more than 10 seconds.

BREATHING

1.) Cover Baby's nose and mouth with your mouth.

2.) Prepare for 2 gentle rescue breaths using the air in your mouth and the strength of your cheeks (not your lungs). Slowly breathe into Baby's mouth for 1 second watching for the chest to rise. If it does, give a second breath, if it doesn't, repeat the head-tilt, chin-lift and try again.

3.) If chest still doesn't rise, examine mouth for foreign objects. If you can see something, swipe it out with your finger. If not, follow first aid for a choking infant.

4.) Begin chest compressions.

CIRCULATION

1.) Imagine a line drawn between the baby's nipples, place two fingers just below that line in the center of the chest.

2.) Gently compress the chest 1/3 to ½ the depth of the chest with two fingers (or encircle chest with hands and push down with thumbs).

3.) Count out loud as you give 30 gentle chest compressions at a rate of about 100-120 per minute.

4.) Give **2 breaths for every 30 chest compressions**.

5.) Perform CPR for 2 minutes before calling for help, unless someone else can call for you.

6.) Continue alternating between two breaths and 30 chest compressions until help arrives.

AIRWAY: TILT HEAD

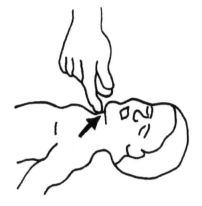

BREATHING: 2 BREATHS

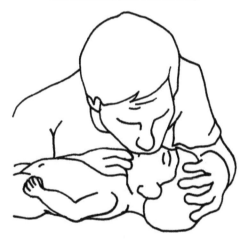

CIRCULATION: 30 CHEST COMPRESSIONS

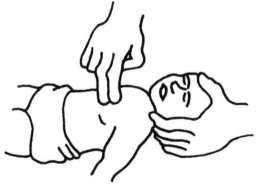

CPR FOR TODDLERS/CHILDREN (12 months – 8 years old)

CPR for toddlers and young children is the same as an infant except the following: 1) use of your hand instead of your fingers for chest compressions, 2) breathe a little deeper, making sure chest rises and, 3) if there is no response after 5 cycles of breathing and chest compressions and an AED (Automated External Defibrillator) is available, apply it and follow prompts using the pediatric pads (if any are in kit). Follow steps below **if there is no response**:

1.) Either have someone call 911 or if you are by yourself, give CPR for 2 minutes before calling for help.
2.) BEGIN the ABC's of CPR: Airway, Breathing and Circulation

AIRWAY (clearing airway)
1.) Place child face up on a firm, flat surface (table or floor is fine).
2.) Tip the head back gently by lifting the chin with one hand and pressing down on the forehead with the other.
3.) Put ear next to child's mouth and listen and look for breathing, for no more than 10 seconds.

BREATHING
1.) Cover child's nose and mouth with your mouth or if child is bigger, clamp their nose with one hand and cover their mouth with your mouth.
2.) Prepare for 2 gentle rescue breaths. Slowly breathe into the child's mouth for 1 second watching for the chest to rise. If it does, give a second breath. If it doesn't, repeat the head-tilt, chin-lift and try again.
3.) If chest still doesn't rise, examine mouth for foreign objects. If you can see something swipe it out with your finger. If not, follow first aid for a choking infant.
4.) Begin chest compressions (below).

CIRCULATION
1.) Imagine a line drawn between the child's nipples, place palm facing down just below that line in the center of the chest.
2.) Gently compress the chest 1/3 to ½ the depth of the chest with the heel of your hand.
3.) Count out loud as you give 30 gentle chest compressions at a rate of about 100-120 per minute.
4.) Give **2 breaths for every 30 chest compressions**.
5.) Perform CPR for 2 minutes before calling 911, unless someone else can call for you.
6.) Continue alternating 2 breaths and 30 chest compressions until help arrives.

AIRWAY: TILT HEAD

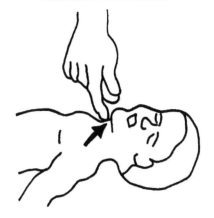

BREATHING: 2 BREATHS

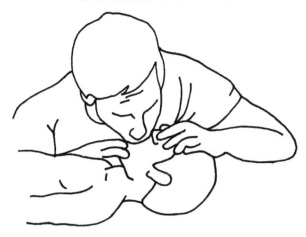

CIRCULATION: 30 CHEST COMPRESSIONS

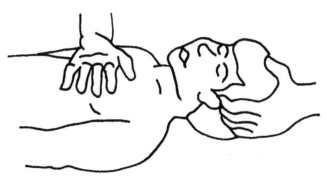

CUTS & SCRAPES (MINOR)

Many babies will get minor cuts and scrapes when they are exploring their environment. These can be easily treated at home. However, if the following occurs, get emergency medical attention:

- Cut is more than ¼" deep or longer than 3"
- Cut has fat or muscle exposed
- You cannot get all debris out of wound

Otherwise, treatment of minor cuts and scrapes is as follows:

1.) Stop the bleeding by applying direct pressure with sterile gauze or clean cloth for 10- 20 minutes.
2.) Clean the wound by rinsing with lots of clean water; make sure all debris is removed. Do not use peroxide. Tweezers sanitized with alcohol can be used.
3.) Apply an antibiotic ointment to wound. If Baby is allergic discontinue.
4.) Cover with a bandage or sterile gauze to keep clean.
5.) Change bandage at least daily or when it becomes dirty or wet.
6.) If the wound ever shows signs of infection: redness around wound, swelling, oozing, or warmth, see the pediatrician.

ELECTRICAL SHOCK

Electrical shock is especially dangerous as many "rescuers" get shocked because they don't understand how electrical current moves.

Call 911 if the following symptoms occur:

- Unconsciousness
- Burn marks where electrical current entered and exited
- Seizures
- Muscles contract or Baby doesn't want to move around

While waiting for help you can:

1.) Look for the electrical current; don't touch anything unless you know the power is off. Never get closer than 20 feet from high-voltage until the power is turned off.
2.) Turn off the source of electricity if possible. If you cannot turn off power and it is not high-voltage, move Baby away from electrical source by using something that is non-conducting, such as cardboard, wood, or plastic.
3.) Don't move Baby, unless in immediate danger.
4.) If Baby isn't breathing, coughing, or moving start CPR.
5.) If able, elevate legs slightly higher than chest to treat shock.

FOREIGN OBJECT IN EYE

Get emergency medical treatment if:
- Object is embedded in eyeball
- Object cannot be removed
- Baby cannot see far away objects or cannot grasp toys (vision blurry)
- Crying after object is removed

What to do in eye emergencies:
1.) Wash hands thoroughly.
2.) Flush eyes with saline solution or clean water liberally and thoroughly. Do not try and wipe foreign body away!
3.) If emergency treatment is needed: cover the eye with an eye cup or tape a plastic cup to the face around the eye so baby doesn't rub or irritate the eye.

NEVER do the following:
- Never rub the eye.
- Never try to remove something embedded in the eyeball.
- Never try to remove a large item that the baby can't close his eye around.

HEAT STROKE

Heat stroke is the most severe of heat-related problems and very dangerous because the body's way of cooling down is not working properly.

If Baby shows any of these symptoms from being overheated, **call 911:**
- Fever: Rectal temperatures greater than:
  - 100.4° F for babies under 3 months of age
  - 101° F for babies 3-6 months of age
  - 103° F for babies 6-12 months of age
  - 104° F for babies over 12 months of age
- Skin hot and dry (could be moist if running/playing)
- No sweating
- Unconscious
- Elevated heartbeat
- Rapid and shallow breathing
- Looks confused, can't walk well (dizzy, lightheaded)
- Nausea

While waiting for medical help, do the following:
1.) Move Baby into a cooler place (shade or air-conditioning). *(continued next page)*

2.) Spray cool, not cold, water on skin, or cover Baby with damp cloths.
3.) Direct air on Baby with a fan or newspaper.
4.) If Baby will drink, give water or if under 6 months of age give formula or breast milk.

HEAD INJURIES / TRAUMA

Many babies fall, hit their head, and do not require medical attention. **But, if any of the following symptoms are present within 15 minutes, call 911:**

- Severe head or facial bleeding
- Seizures
- Bleeding from the nose or ears
- Change in level of consciousness for more than a few seconds
- Vomiting
- Bruising below eyes or behind ears
- Loss of balance
- Weakness or an inability to use an arm or leg
- Unequal pupil size
- Slurred speech, or difference in babbling

If Baby does show any of the signs above, while waiting for medical attention do the following:

1.) Keep Baby as still as possible in a dark room with shoulders/head elevated. **Avoid moving Baby**, especially the neck area, if at all possible.
2.) Put pressure on any bleeding to slow, but avoid if the skull may be fractured.
3.) If Baby shows no signs of movement, coughing, or breathing, start CPR.

If none of the above symptoms are seen within 15 minutes, there should be no cause for real concern.

INSECT BITES / STINGS

Most insect bites and stings are considered minor with just an annoying itch or sting at the injection site.

However, if the following symptoms are present, call 911:
- Facial, throat, or lip swelling
- Difficulty breathing
- Abdominal pain (crying and holding stomach)
- Dizziness
- Elevated heart beat
- Hives
- Vomiting or bleeding from the mouth
- Not acting normal, seeming confused, or disoriented
- Inconsolable crying for more than 5-10 minutes

If severe, do the following while waiting for medical help:
1.) Loosen clothing and cover with blanket – do not swaddle!
2.) Do not give anything to drink.
3.) If vomiting or bleeding from the mouth, lie on side to avoid choking.
4.) Try to calm the baby, hold horizontal with feet raised slightly above head.
5.) If breathing stops, start CPR.

If the sting or bite is minor, treat at home by doing the following:
1.) Move to a safer area to avoid more stings or bites.
2.) Scrape off the stinger with a straight-edged object such as a credit card or back of a knife.
3.) Apply ice pack; do not apply ice directly to the skin.
4.) If over 6 months of age, apply hydrocortisone cream (.5% or 1%), calamine lotion, or baking soda paste (three teaspoons soda to one teaspoon water) to infected area several times a day – cover with gauze if using creams.
5.) **NOTE:** Do not use topical Benadryl or any topical anti-histamine that contains diphenhydramine because they give immediate relief but can cause rebound symptoms that are worse.
   If under 6 months of age, apply only baking soda paste several times a day.
6.) If over 6 months of age and continues to itch or swell, Benadryl (diphenhydramine) syrup by mouth can be given.

POISONING
Always call 911 or Poison Control Center Hotline 800-222-1222.

Never give anything by mouth until instructed to do so. Product labels may contain wrong information so consult a professional and do not follow the label.

While waiting for help, immediately do the following:
- If poison is in eyes: immediately flush with water for 15-20 minutes.
- If poison is inhaled: get to fresh air immediately.
- If poison is on the skin: take off any clothing with poison and rinse with water for 15-20 minutes.

PUNCTURE WOUND
These wounds can be dangerous because they can easily get infected. Punctures from an animal bite or on the foot are at even greater risk of getting infected.

Get immediate medical attention if:
- Puncture deep enough to draw blood and doesn't stop after a couple minutes
- Pieces of debris cannot be removed
- Animal bites that pierce skin (most need to be treated with antibiotics)

If there is no bleeding or bleeding is minimal, do the following:
1.) Stop the bleeding by applying pressure directly to wound.
2.) Rinse or clean with water, make sure all pieces of debris/material are removed from wound.
3.) Apply antibiotic ointment to decrease the risk of infection; if Baby has a reaction to the ointment, discontinue.
4.) Cover the wound with sterile gauze or a bandage.
5.) If Baby has never had a tetanus vaccine, one needs to be administered within 48 hours; call the pediatrician.
6.) Change the bandage regularly and every time it gets wet.
7.) If the wound ever shows signs of infection: redness around wound, swelling, oozing, or warmth, call the pediatrician.

Report any animal that has uncontrollable behavior or has rabies.

SEVERE BLEEDING

If internal bleeding is suspected, especially from a fall or collision, call 911. Internal bleeding symptoms are:

- Bleeding from ears, nose, mouth, rectum, or vagina
- Vomiting or coughing blood
- Wounds that are on the skull, chest, or abdomen
- Bruising on neck, chest, abdomen, or side (between ribs)
- Bone fractures
- Cries when you touch their abdomen or abdomen muscles spasm when touched
- Skin turns cool to touch, indicating onset of shock

Follow these steps:

1.) Wash hands, if possible, before touching to decrease risk of infection.
2.) Lay Baby on ground with legs and bleeding area slightly elevated, if possible. **Do not move them** if injury to spine or neck is suspected.
3.) Remove any large surface debris.
4.) If any organs are misplaced/removed, do not try to put them back or arrange them.
5.) Apply direct pressure on the wound preferably with a sterile bandage but a clean cloth, towel, or bare hand will work for at least 20 minutes.
6.) If bleeding is massive or doesn't reduce after 15 minutes, call 911 or emergency help – but do not remove pressure bandage!
7.) If pressure cloth gets saturated with blood, do not remove, just add more cloth and continue holding.
8.) Once bleeding has stopped, leave pressure cloths in place and take to emergency room.

SHOCK

Shock can happen for a variety of reasons and is extremely serious. **If any of the following symptoms are present, call 911:**

- Skin is cool and clammy
- Skin is pale or gray
- Elevated heartbeat but weak pulse
- Breathing slow and shallow, or heavy and fast (hyperventilation)
- Pupils dilated and Baby staring or looking as though daydreaming
- Baby can be conscious or unconscious *(continued next page)*

Things to do while waiting for help:
1.) Keep Baby as still as possible. Either hold horizontally or lay flat on his or her side.
2.) Elevate the legs, if possible, without causing more injury.
3.) If Baby isn't moving, coughing, or breathing, start CPR.
4.) Loosen any tight clothing.
5.) Cover with a light blanket.
6.) Do not give any liquids or food.

SUNBURN

Sunburns in infants can sometimes be more serious than parents may think. Call the pediatrician if the following occurs:

- Blisters within 24 hours
- Over 4" in diameter
- Fever over 100.4° F for under 1 month of age
- Fever over 101° F for 1-3 months of age
- Fever over 103° F for ages over 3 months of age

Minor sunburns (those not having any of the above symptoms) can be treated at home following these steps:
1.) Make sure Baby gets enough fluids.
2.) Soak a flannel, terry, or muslin cloth in cool water and place on burn for 15 minutes a few times a day – especially right after being exposed.
3.) Bathe Baby in a lukewarm bath with a teaspoon of baking soda.
4.) Apply water based lotions, aloe-vera gel, or calamine lotion for relief.
5.) DO NOT USE petroleum-based gels, lotions, or ointments as these can worsen the burn by trapping the heat and sweat.
6.) Avoid re-exposure to sun until burn heals.
7.) Can administer acetaminophen if pediatrician recommends.

Note: Sunscreen, at least SPF 30, should *ALWAYS* be used when a baby is exposed to sunlight outdoors. Babies under 6 months of age should never be exposed to direct sunlight. Sunscreen labels state not to use if a baby is less than 6 months because they should not be in the sun at all.

TICK BITE

If a tick bites Baby, follow these steps:

1.) Disinfect the area around the tick bite with alcohol or rinse with water.

2.) Remove the tick as soon as possible with a pair of tweezers. The longer you wait, the harder it is to remove. Be sure to carefully squeeze the head and gently pull. Do not separate the head and body.

3.) Save the tick in a sealed jar if possible. Later, if Baby has a reaction the doctor can use it for analysis.

4.) Thoroughly wash your hands, the area around the tick bite, and any skin that came in contact with the tick with soap and water.

If any of the following symptoms are present, call 911:

- Inconsolable crying
- Difficulty breathing or seems out of breath
- Doesn't move
- Irregular heart rhythm

Baby needs to see the pediatrician if all of the tick cannot be removed or if any of these symptoms are present:

- Fever
- Rash
- Decreased movement
- Swollen lymph nodes
- Stiff neck
- Flu-like symptoms

PERSONAL NOTES

BABYSITTER CHECKLIST

Leave and review the following information with a babysitter.
(This can be copied and posted.)

Eat and Sleep Schedule

_____

_____

_____

_____

_____

Food While Away (note any allergies)

_____

_____

_____

Medications (times & dosages)

_____

_____

Bedtime (time & routine)

_____

_____

Other Instructions

_____

_____

Parent Location & Phone # _____

Alternate Phone #_____

Neighbor Name & Phone # _____

Approximate Time Back _____

Review posted emergency phone numbers and information page, fire
emergency plans, and where babysitter is allowed to take baby (if
anywhere other than inside home).

EMERGENCY PHONE NUMBERS & INFO

(Copy and post by the phone. Update regularly.)

Parents:

Name _____

Work # _____ Cell #_____

Name _____

Work # _____ Cell #_____

House Address _____

Relative Name & # _____

Neighbor Name & # _____

Pediatrician:

Name _____

Office # _____ Nurse Line# _____

Baby:

Birth Date_____

Allergies (food & medications)

_____

Current Medications _____

_____

Poison Control Center   **1-800-222-1222**

Fire Department _____
Police Department _____

National Domestic Violence   **1-800-799-SAFE** (7233)
Hotline (24 hrs/day)   1-800-878-3224 TTY for deaf

CPSIA information can be obtained
at www.ICGtesting.com
Printed in the USA
BVHW07s0817210818
524968BV00002B/213/P

9 781608 444458